I'LL DO IT TOMORROW

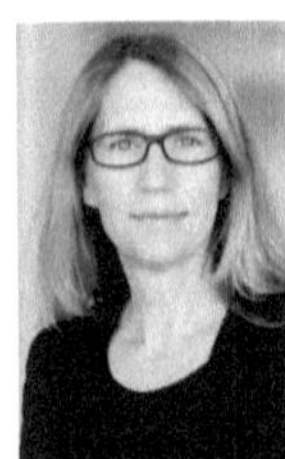

HELLE FOLDEN DYBDAHL

Chief psychologist.
Helle is a specialist in work and organisational psychology. She has worked as an industrial psychologist for years, focusing on strategic management, prevention and managing stress and other mental health disorders at employee, managerial and organisational level.

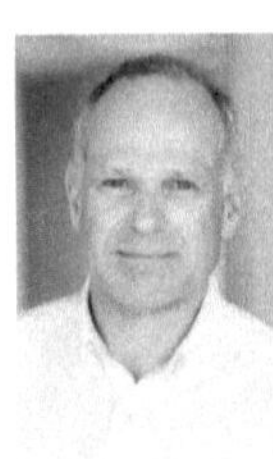

JESPER KARLE

Consultant in psychiatry, MD, Dr Med
Jesper has in-depth expertise in psychiatric investigation and treatment having researched and taught extensively. Moreover, he has co-authored numerous articles within the fields of psychiatry and neuroscience.

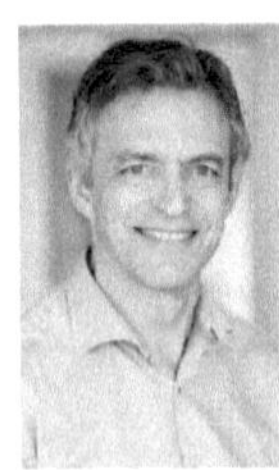

LARS AAKERLUND

Consultant in psychiatry, MD, PhD.
Lars has worked with psychiatric treatment and counselling for years, has taught in numerous private and public organisations and has co-authored several articles.

HELLE FOLDEN DYBDAHL

JESPER KARLE

LARS AAKERLUND

I'LL DO IT TOMORROW

4 STEPS TO STRESS PREVENTION MANAGEMENT

PPPUBLISHERS

Professional, insightful, simple and well-written. One of the best and most balanced books I've read about stress and stress prevention. Anyone with just the slightest bit of managerial responsibility should read it.

★ ★ ★ ★ ★
Søren Strunk-Sørensen, InsideBusiness

This book takes the manager by the hand as it explains, and illustrates through examples, what can be at stake for overwhelmed employees and how managers can tackle situations where employees are beginning to show signs of being under pressure. A book that is guaranteed to prevent more stress-related sick leave than more legislation and control from the authorities will.
Great inspiration for the manager who wants to prevent stress developing among their employees.

★ ★ ★ ★ ★
Signe Tønnesen, Senior consultant, the Danish Association of Managers and Executives, Altinget

Between stimulus and response there is a space.
In that space is our power to choose our response.
In our response lies our growth and our freedom.

Viktor E. Frankl

I'll do it tomorrow
4 steps to stress prevention management
Helle Folden Dybdahl, Jesper Karle and Lars Aakerlund
© 2019 Helle Folden Dybdahl, Jesper Karle and Lars Aakerlund
Original Danish title:
Jeg gør det i morgen
Fra undgåelse til stressforebyggende ledelse
Helle Folden Dybdahl, Jesper Karle and Lars Aakerlund
© 2018 Helle Folden Dybdahl, Jesper Karle and Lars Aakerlund
English translation © 2019 Sinéad Quirke Køngerskov

Cover, layout and illustrations: Klahr
Editing: Mette de Fine Licht and Heidi Korsgaard, Skriveværkstedet
Proofreading: Jane Davis
Printed by: Fjerritslev Tryk

ISBN: 978-87-970865-1-3

1st edition 2019

CONTENTS

BREAK THE STRESS CURVE

IN 4 STEPS

What if we could lead a busy life without it making us sick? What if we were able to deal with the challenges that life throws at us, whether it be overtime, divorce or something else, without it having to lead to taking sick leave? What if we could slow down the development of stress-related disorders such as anxiety and depression? And what if everyone could experience a better work day? A work day with wellbeing and a shared focus on dealing with challenges as they arise and before they develop into even bigger problems and stress.

We believe it is possible!

We can't promise that we can remove all the discomfort and pressure of everyday life – that's a part of being human – but, through this book, we share our inspiration for how we can help each other create a life where the challenges we face at home and at work don't have to develop into stress and disease.

For the past 17 years, we've been working intensively with both the treatment and prevention of stress. We have advised leaders, managers and employees across Europe and all types of organisations – both public and private – and we were behind a PhD on the subject (ref. 1). As a psychologist and medical specialists within the field of stress and stress-related disorders, we have talked to people with all kinds of and at all stages of stress-related disorders. We've learned that the sooner a person receives the right help to deal with stress, the less effort is needed and the better the result. We have also gained insight into the early stages of stress development, which, in turn, caused us to develop an interest in the very early prevention of stress. Today, we know that much can be done quite early on to prevent a person developing dangerous stress symptoms. This is what is new in our book; what we collectively call stress prevention management.

Some parts of the book are supported by research, while other parts are based on experience and case stories. Through these we present our ideas for how we can work together to break the stress curve, starting with leadership and management in the workplace. Not just in theory but in practice too.

> "It's not enough to have knowledge on stress and an opinion of stress. Real stress prevention requires the right action at the right time."

Our places of work are often berated for being the cause of people's stress, while our managers and leaders are the scapegoated group who needs to stop tyrannising employees. But workplaces have to understand that employees need safeguarding.

We believe it's neither reasonable nor constructive to demonise managers or employers or to lay all the blame and responsibility on them. We meet many managers who want to reduce stress among their employees, but who find it difficult to do so. Because what are you supposed to do as a manager – and what should you avoid?

As you read this book, you'll see that we understand stress as something to be dealt with collectively. Places of employment and managers are a central part of the solution for an employee experiencing stress – even if the symptoms of stress aren't from the pressures of work, but are due to other conditions in the workplace or challenges in their personal life.

Our goal with this book is to provide you, as a manager, with an understanding of how you can help prevent a lack of thriving and dissatisfaction among your employees, and how you can stop early signs of stress from developing into more severe stress, disease and sick leave. It's not just about doing "something" as a manager. With this book, we take that further and present what we believe you need to know about both your employees and yourself, and how, as a manager, you can contribute to preventing stress through your management and leadership.

Debunking myths about stress

Our aim with this book is also to challenge and point out the nuances in the current perception of stress. Despite the publication of numerous good books and articles on stress, many myths about what stress is and how best to treat it abound. These myths mean that much of the efforts aimed at targeting stress in organisations and companies are built on an outdated and rigid view of stress. Some little effect may, of course, be seen, but we don't *really* get any further. We would like to change that.

Every day, 35,000 people in Denmark alone take sick leave due to stress and stress-related disorders, such as anxiety and depression. And a probably even larger number goes to work while showing symptoms of stress, not feeling or doing well and performing badly at work – what is termed "presenteeism". It's hard for them, their families and their places of work. And losing so much of the labour force is a huge loss for society. Many of those who are absent due to stress never return to the work market, which was precisely what we addressed in our first book, *Tag på arbejde – fra sygemelding til samarbejde [Go to Work – From Sick Note to Fit Note* – available in Danish*]* (2016). In it, we focused on how the various parties involved, including employers, get people back to work after they have been absent due to illness. Now we want to avoid sick leave in the first place. In other words, our mission with this book is to make our first book redundant.

You need to challenge your avoidance behaviour

For years, we've been allowed to listen to and help people who have been affected by lesser or more severe symptoms of stress.

It's experience from these conversations that forms the basis of the examples presented here. However, as this is a book about preventing and taking early action on stress, many of the stories don't bear the mark of people who have been suffering for a long time. Rather the stories are about people who are in such early phases of stress that neither they nor their managers necessarily know they are dealing with the early onset of stress. That's how it starts for most people. The stories are real and have been taken from our work with employees with stress and from our discussions with managers. All personal details have been changed.

You will notice that the people you meet in this book rarely develop symptoms of stress from *too much work* alone. There's usually much more than piles of papers putting pressure on them. Common to all of them is that those who do best discuss their experience of being weighed down with stress early on with their managers. And they work with their managers on finding concrete solutions, which prevent symptoms of stress from developing.

And it's precisely this collaboration between employees and managers, with the aim of avoiding the development of symptoms of stress, that we focus on here. A collaboration, which, as a manager and leader, you can take responsibility for creating through a targeted focus on stress prevention management.

You may think there isn't much new in that, because you already talk to your employees. But do you still talk to them when they first begin to withdraw from you too? Or when they get angry with you? The key issue is for you to understand that you have to challenge your avoidance behaviour. You have to be willing to learn to face problems and to talk to your employees in a way that few people are used to. The goal is to learn to be professionally curious rather than waiting to see what happens or avoiding what is hard due to a fear of getting too close, being too personal or making the situation worse.

Mental issues are rarely easy to work with, but the tools we give you here are quite simple in principle. Though they can be challenging to put into practice, at least in the beginning. You may have to let go of some habits and adopt a few new ones. You might also have to draw up a new basic perception of stress. But you will find over time that stress-related sick leave in your organisation will decline.

We can't guarantee that you will never have to call in a temp, send a get well card or take a sick day yourself if you start practising the four steps that are at the heart of stress prevention management. But if you use the book's methods, you will need fewer temps in the future. And employee job satisfaction will increase. This is how we can break the stress curve together – with the workplace as the starting point for prevention.

The book is primarily for those who are managers and leaders, but we would recommend that you share what we write here with your employees.

Happy Reading,

Helle Folden Dybdahl, Jesper Karle and Lars Aakerlund
2019

STRESS PREVENTION MANAGEMENT

People are different and react differently
to the same events.

Much of what creates stress for the individual
can be removed or significantly reduced.

It's important to create space and conditions
so that each employee can be helped at an
early stage with practical solutions to bring
them back to an experience of being in
control of their own life.

WHAT DO WE KNOW ABOUT STRESS AND HOW CAN WE PREVENT IT?

Newspapers often write about stress. Magazines feature articles with advice from stress experts. And bookshelves overflow with books on stress – including one we've written in addition to this volume. So why yet another book about stress? We'd like to answer that question by asking another question: has it helped? Has the number of people experiencing stress reduced?

The short answer is: no. According to the Danish Health Authority (ref. 2), in 2007, 9 per cent of the Danish population often experienced being stressed. Seven years later, in 2014, the figure had risen to 15 per cent. In other words, every sixth Dane often felt stressed. And this sad development has continued in recent years. According to the Danish Health Authority's figures for 2017, 25 per cent of the population experienced a high level of stress and 19 per cent of employed Danes felt very stressed. But it's even worse for those who aren't in work – as many as 47 per cent of them are living with a high level of stress. This figure suggests that it's not only our workload that can make us stressed. We'll return to this later.

HOW STRESSED ARE THE DANES?

2007:
- 9 % of the Danish population experience that they often feel stressed.

2014:
- 15 % of the Danish population experience that they often feel stressed.

2017:
- 25 % of the Danish population experience a high level of stress.

And, if we turn to our European neighbours, a 2018 study by the Mental Health Foundation of 4,619 British respondents – the largest known study of stress levels in the UK to date – found that a staggering 74 per cent of those polled had felt so stressed over the previous year that they had felt overwhelmed or unable to cope, with women reporting more stress than men (ref. 3). While, further across the pond, a 2014 online survey by the American Psychological Association thankfully found that the number of Americans saying stress has impacted their physical or mental health (25 per cent in 2015 vs 37 per cent in 2011 and 28 per cent in 2014 vs 35 per cent in 2011, respectively) is declining. Yet, 75 per cent of the 3,068 Americans polled reported experiencing at least one physical symptom of stress in the past month, with parents, women, younger generations and those living in low-income households reporting higher levels of stress overall (ref. 4). These figures are alarming, even allowing for differences in population, because despite the fact that we talk and write so much about stress, the number of people who are stressed is growing. And the issue is that we aren't building a bridge between the theories of stress and effective stress prevention in practice. Nowadays, we know a lot about what creates wellbeing and job satisfaction. We also know that there is an important relationship between severe stress and some well-defined disorders, such as depression and anxiety. And yet we haven't found the answer to limiting stress.

The media tends to have a particular focus on stress. Five repeated messages are:

1) Stress is dangerous.
2) Stress is a physical disease.
3) Stress is being in a state of overload.
4) Stress demands peace and calm.
5) Stress is a diagnosis.

The commonly accepted definition of stress reads: "a special relationship between the person and the environment, which is perceived as a strain on the person or which exceeds his or her resources and threatens his or her wellbeing" (ref. 5). This is a broad definition, which covers many different problems. But what do we actually know about stress? What facts do we have? Let's get something straight right away: stress is neither a specific condition nor a medical diagnosis. The word "stress" is used indiscriminately and as a term for everything from mild symptoms to severe diseases requiring specific treatment. If we look at the diagnostic manual ICD-10 (International Classification of Disorder – 10th Edition) by the World Health Organisation

(WHO), stress doesn't feature at all as a diagnosis. In ICD-10, there are diagnoses of stress-related conditions in the form of "adjustment disorders", "acute stress reaction" and "post-traumatic stress disorder". These conditions are triggered by external strain. And there are diagnoses for disorders such as "anxiety disorders" and "depression" – disorders that can be wholly or partially stress-related. But pure "stress" as a diagnosis isn't included.

According to WHO, in just a few years stress-related depression will be the most widespread epidemic. When we encounter people who have been labelled as "stressed", many of them are suffering from diseases such as depression or anxiety disorders, while other people's symptoms are mild and transient and pass once the strain comes to an end.

The *symptoms* of stress can be both physical and mental. And they can be severe. If you have been on sick leave with a stress-related health problem, or if you know someone who has, you know that the symptoms felt in relation to stress can be very unpleasant and feel quite threatening. The symptoms are real and they can make you sick if you don't intervene in time.

If you believe that stress is a clearly defined and distinctly demarcated disorder triggered by external (over)burdening, then you probably also believe that proper treatment exists. And for most people that equates to peace and quiet. We find it worrying that this is how the majority still understand stress. We don't disagree that you may need peace and quiet and a shorter period of sick leave if you experience severe symptoms of stress. But stress is much more nuanced than that and can, as we mentioned above, cover a large number of different conditions. If you talk to a group of people who are all experiencing serious stress, it will manifest itself in each of them quite differently. On the one hand are people with severe stress-related diseases, particularly depression and anxiety disorders. And on the other are people who don't feel well, but who haven't developed a disorder and who, therefore, don't need to be diagnosed with anything at all.

In our experience, peace and quiet isn't the only treatment effective for people who are considered to be severely stressed, and every day we see the unfortunate consequences of long-term sick leave, in stressed people who become increasingly ill. Peace and quiet may – perhaps – dull the symptoms of stress for a while and can put a lid on some worries, negative thoughts and the experience of discomfort, but peace and quiet also risk the same thoughts, feelings and physical discomfort being exacerbated. Thus, as we wrote about in our first book, the person's health risks deteriorating still further if creating a sustainable solution isn't tackled early on in the process.

Because stress arises for many different reasons, we should prevent and manage stress with different individual solutions too, depending on what the individual is experiencing. This is one of the crucial points of this book – that, as a manager and leader, you should take an interest in the individual person's experience early on, so you can avoid a lack of attention and action worsening the symptoms of stress and leading to serious illness.

In our view, the workplace is the best starting point for seriously reducing widespread stress. We mean this – despite many people believing this is actually where all the stress stems from and that work is a place to get away from in order to get rid of stress. If we can recognise and accept that stress requires an interest in the individual person and we start working from there, we can go far.

Exactly how far was revealed in a 2014 British guide, which showed the positive results of three major British companies after they had introduced programmes for dealing with mental health problems, including stress (ref. 6). Here, managers took early action and various employee initiatives were implemented in workplaces, so employees weren't simply sent home on sick leave when they experienced stress or mental health issues. Absence due to illness caused by psychological problems and stress complaints dropped dramatically at all three companies, by up to 50 per cent, and at one company alone, the savings in relation to sick leave were calculated to be the equivalent of £1.3 million. Such a huge sum begs the question: can we afford not to do anything? According to another British report from 2017 (ref. 7), 40 per cent of all sickness absence is due to stress, anxiety and depression.

Only the cost of sick leave related to mental health was calculated here. An even bigger problem is the phenomenon of presenteeism, which means reduced productivity due to going to work while presenting with symptoms of stress. A British government report from 2012 (ref. 8) estimates that the social cost of presenteeism is 2.6 times greater than that caused by absence due to illness. There is so much to gain from early intervention and from helping people avoid getting sick.

A nuanced view of stress

If we really want to understand stress and develop solid methods to prevent it, then we need to challenge the myths and develop a nuanced understanding of stress. Stress *can* be a phenomenon of overburdening that develops as a response to too much work, as many people currently believe. But this isn't necessarily the case. We should understand stress, to a much greater extent, as an individual intellectual and emotional reaction to *experienced* strain – a reaction that can occur as a result of many different reasons. This is why we can never break the stress curve with a one-size-fits-all solution, such as reducing workload or hours, improving the employee's overall health or moving the employee away from the workplace. We need to be interested in the individual person's experience and interpretation; that is, the thoughts and feelings they have about the strain they are experiencing.

IMPORTANT TO KNOW ABOUT STRESS

- Stress is a normal reaction that all human beings can develop.
- Stress is an intellectual and emotional reaction to something a person experiences as difficult or as a burden or strain.
- The burden may be due to work, but it can also be caused by something else entirely.
- Stress can be related to workload, but certainly not always.
- Given that stress isn't always due to too much work, then neither can stress always be cured by reducing the workload or seeking out peace and quiet.
- Experiencing short-term symptoms of stress is a natural part of being human and isn't dangerous. We shouldn't be afraid of stress symptoms, but should rather ensure they don't persist and worsen.
- Shielding an employee with early stress symptoms by isolating them from the working community can aggravate the situation.
- The symptoms of stress are both mental and physical. Stress can lead to mental and/or physical illness.
- Prevention works if we focus on the individual's *experience and interpretation* of the burden and the symptoms.
- Prevention works if we step in when the symptoms begin – not if they have developed into a disorder. Symptoms often start with a feeling of dissatisfaction due to a change or an experience of unfairness.
- The workplace is part of the solution, regardless of whether the cause of the stress symptoms is in the individual's work or private life.
- As a manager, you should intervene when an employee shows signs of stress – even if you think their stress is due to something in their private life.

Stress models

There are a number of models that try to explain when we develop stress. Some models focus on which external factors can trigger stress among employees at work. Other models focus on how employees perceive and understand factors that trigger stress. According to the Danish Working Environment Authority, three of the major models are the demand-control model, the effort-reward model and the job demand-resource model (ref. 9). The starting point of all three models is stress due to the imbalance between the demands placed on an employee at work and the opportunities the employee has for dealing with those demands.

STRESS MODELS
- Demand-control model: an employee can feel stressed when they face high demands on the job and at the same time have little influence on their work duties. Perhaps several tasks have to be done by a short deadline (high demand), but they can't say no to new tasks (little influence).
- Effort-reward model: an employee can feel stressed when they experience an imbalance between the effort they make in their work and the reward they receive.
- Job demand-resource model: an employee can feel stressed when they experience an imbalance between the demands of work and their own resources. Resources could, for example, be support from the management or team of colleagues.

The Danish Working Environment Authority states that, taken together, these models cover the following important points:

- Job-related stress can occur when there is an imbalance between burden and resources.
- There may be different types of imbalance in different jobs.
- There is a difference between how we experience burdens and interpret resources. What stresses one employee won't necessarily stress their colleague.

Here, the three classic stress models are correct. We do indeed see a lot of people who work a certain number of hours and have demands placed on them that obviously exceed their resources, which, in turn, leads to symptoms of stress and disease. But the models are far from adequate. We are now seeing even more people who find that the demands being made of them are unmanageable, but whom, when *seen objectively,* aren't burdened. This doesn't change the person's own experience of feeling under pressure. And so we are back to the disparity that exists between the objective image and the person's own experience, and which it's necessary to shine a light on in order to move forward with the prevention of more serious stress.

In the 1960s, attempts were made to award points to different types of stress in order to compare the severity of the burden (ref. 10). For example, points were given if you were dismissed from your job, got a new job or got divorced. The idea was that by counting up the points you could see who was stressed and who wasn't. But some of those awarded the most points had no symptoms of stress at all. And some people who got very few points had many symptoms. One or many external strains don't necessarily indicate who will react with symptoms of stress and who won't.

So if we are going to understand when we are likely to respond with symptoms of stress, we need a more nuanced understanding of stress as a reaction stemming from thoughts and emotions. External burdens don't necessarily lead to a stress reaction. And a stress reaction can come about without any external strain. It all depends on the individual person's *experience and interpretation of the situation*. And this is a question of three elements:

* Burden/strain
* The individual interpretation
* Reaction

From burden to reaction

Let's take a closer look at "the three-part model", which can offer a good foundation for effectively preventing stress as it breaks with the traditional perception of stress. The model shows that it's not just about looking at or removing the burden from the employee. It's just as much about taking an interest in the individual employee's experience and interpretation of the situation. Let's look at an example of how an employee can experience a job assignment in two very different ways and experience completely different degrees of pressure in relation to it.

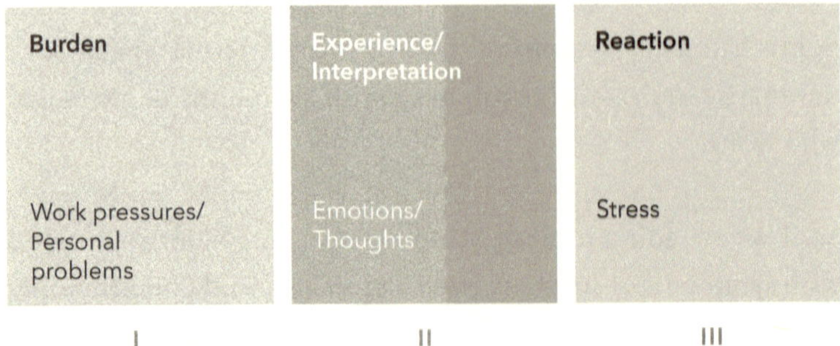

The three-part model

You go to one of your employees and tell them about a huge, new project, for which they are going to be the lead. It's complex and important, but the parameters aren't quite clear yet. Your employee can respond in two ways:

A: "Oh no, what I hear my boss saying is that I alone am going to be responsible for the success of the project. I'll have to find a way to do it and all my other work at the same time. My boss expects me to be able to do it – otherwise she wouldn't have given me the job. If I can't do it, I'll disappoint her and who knows, maybe they won't be able to use me here anymore."

B: "It's a complex but exciting project. My boss has asked me to take the lead, so I'll have to try to take the first steps and get an overview of the project. If it gets too difficult for me, I'll have to ask for help from my boss or colleagues. I'll have to work out how much time I'm going to need to spend on it, so I know what other jobs I can't do, and then I'll have to talk to my boss about it."

Note that the project – the objective burden – is the same. But the experience and interpretation of the situation is very different. The example demonstrates that stress prevention doesn't necessarily lie in removing the job at hand, but in examining how the individual employee *experiences and interprets* the assignments they get.

A fruit basket isn't enough

Given the importance of taking an interest in the individual employee's experience and interpretation, which we have just described, it is, of course, problematic that so many people equate prevention with general health and wellbeing.

Many of the initiatives for preventing stress that are currently gaining ground are based on a broad and unspecific approach to employee welfare. There is much well-meaning advice on eating healthily, exercising, getting plenty of sleep and disconnecting with mindfulness. And, on the face of it, the easy and practical advice has also – to a large extent – become the pivotal point of research in relation to creating a good working environment. Indeed, "the 6 pearls of wisdom" have long provided a framework for how to prevent stress in the workplace.

THE 6 PEARLS OF WISDOM:
- Influence
- Social support
- Reward
- Predictability
- Purpose
- Demand.

Source: The Danish National Research Centre for the Working Environment (ref. 11)

Many places of employment would like to support their employees' health; fruit baskets, organic canteens, massages and gym memberships are provided for employees. Some workplaces are even trying to help employees improve their sleep patterns. Others arrange after-work meetings on "the healthy working environment". Fruit baskets, fitness and after-work meetings are definitely good initiatives if you want to develop and maintain a good workplace and help employees have a healthy lifestyle. But if we want to reduce stress and absence due to illness, we can't focus on the general health of employees alone. Free fruit and after-work meetings don't prevent or eliminate the reaction that arises in each of us when we experience pressure or an unwelcome change, or when we feel misunderstood or unfairly treated. And they certainly don't help the employee who is experiencing a concrete, pressurised situation and who needs their manager's help in resolving it.

Whose fault is it?

Paradoxically, the much well-intentioned advice on exercise, diet, sleep and effective working days can actually – despite the best intentions – make us even more stressed, because the responsibility for our wellbeing at work and job satisfaction has now become our own. If we develop stress, it's our own fault. To have avoided it, we should simply have followed some of the many suggestions.

Many people also point to the employee themselves being to blame for the stress. It can be just as wrong to blame the individual employee for stress as it is to blame their place of work.

There are, of course, exceptions to this. Some workplaces contribute to creating stress among a large group of employees; for example, by the workload exceeding what the employees can manage. There are also managers who have an adverse and stress-inducing effect on their employees. And yes, there are employees who are at particular personal risk of developing stress, employees who have difficulty taking care of themselves and employees who are poorly suited to the job they are in. And, lastly, we sometimes see collaboration problems and general dissatisfaction with the job being "masked" as stress. All of this helps confuse the picture.

That said, we actually have to get away from placing blame. Instead, we have to recognise that stress prevention at work needs to be based on the relationship between you as a manager and your employee; that is, the one to one relationship. This can be a crucial starting point for breaking the stress curve.

As it stands today, many managers fail to intervene at the first signs of stress. Perhaps you know this from your own personal experience. You avoid talking to an employee about what is putting them under pressure, for fear they will reveal something you can't handle. Or you are afraid that you'll get too close and become involved in something personal. This may be related to the nature of stress itself – stress includes anxiety, and anxiety is at the heart of avoidance behaviour. And avoiding what is difficult ends up applying to both you and your employee.

New prevention methods

There's a disconnect between what we today call the prevention of stress – for example, all the many health initiatives – and the help given to the individual employee who has become stressed or ill. In other words, there is a "missing link" between the organisation's health initiatives and the treatment of the individual employee, for example, by a psychologist.

If we want to put an end to stress, we need to focus precisely on the point at which symptoms of stress haven't yet developed into a disorder that will require treatment. Rather we need to focus on where the employee is clearly experiencing pressure and needs assistance through leadership and management to get better because the general health initiatives within the organisation aren't sufficient and they can't handle the feelings of dissatisfaction and discontent on their own.

The missing link

Organisation

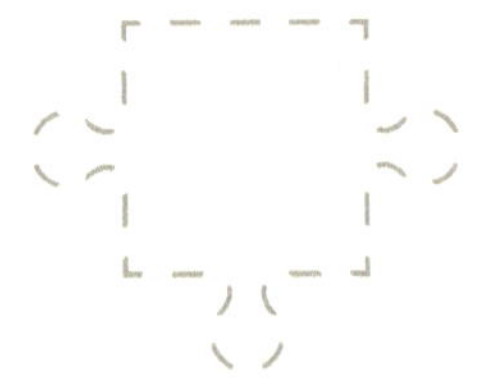

Psykolog

This is when the employee needs leadership – what we call stress prevention management. This is where you have to step in and be **professionally curious** about your employee.

Professional curiosity involves you as a manager and leader:

- Being aware of behavioural changes in each employee, particularly small changes that may be the first signs of stress.
- Asking questions so you and your employee come to a common understanding of what is at stake for them.
- Helping your employee with a solution that brings them back to a place of control.
- Following up with frequent conversations about their wellbeing.

You may be wondering why this should be part of your role. As a manager and leader, it's your job to *lead* your employees – even when it's difficult. You are the one out in front, showing how your workplace tackles challenges. As a manager, you have a responsibility to your place of employment, the group and the individual employee.

With regard to work duties – that is, the task you and your employees are employed to resolve – and the group's wellbeing, as the manager, you have a particular responsibility for the employees experiencing that you can work together, that things happen fairly, that you are trustworthy and that the employees can trust each other. One of the most destructive things for a group's wellbeing are employees who are affected by – and possibly on sick leave with – stress. This typically destabilises the group's experience of its ability to collaborate and of fairness as well as the level of trust within the group. And that has consequences for the common purpose: the task at hand (ref. 11).

When it comes to the individual employee, as the manager, you have a responsibility for ensuring that they get the help and support they need. Thus, you have a responsibility to investigate what help is needed and find a possible solution if an employee is experiencing being under pressure and feeling challenged. As a manager, you have a responsibility not to avoid the problem, but to face it head on.

If managers need to be aware of the work, the group's wellbeing and the individual employee, then stress prevention is absolutely central.

There is nothing new in managers having to talk to their employees. Our message is for you to be aware of *what* you are talking to your employees about and *when* you talk to them. Stress prevention management is largely about thinking differently and not withdrawing or avoiding taking action – something we can all be inclined to do when someone is having difficulty. In Step 2 we give you solid, practical advice on how to develop and work with professional curiosity. And we acknowledge that being a manager is demanding and entails a number of difficult challenges. So bear with us if we sometimes seem to simplify things in this book. We aren't in any way trying to make things sound easier than they are in real life.

Go after what actions are available

Serious stress-related disorders, such as depression and anxiety, don't occur because an employee has had a few bad days. Or because they have been sleeping badly for a while. They typically develop over time, often several months. And you can very often avoid that development by identifying it and tackling it as early as possible.

In the figure, you can see what options are available to you, as a manager, in relation to an employee developing stress. The earlier in the process you step in, the greater the opportunity you have to help. And vice versa – the later you intervene, the harder it will be for you to do something for your employee and help them get back on track as the employee will increasingly need health care, i.e. psychological and/or medical treatment. This process limits your options.

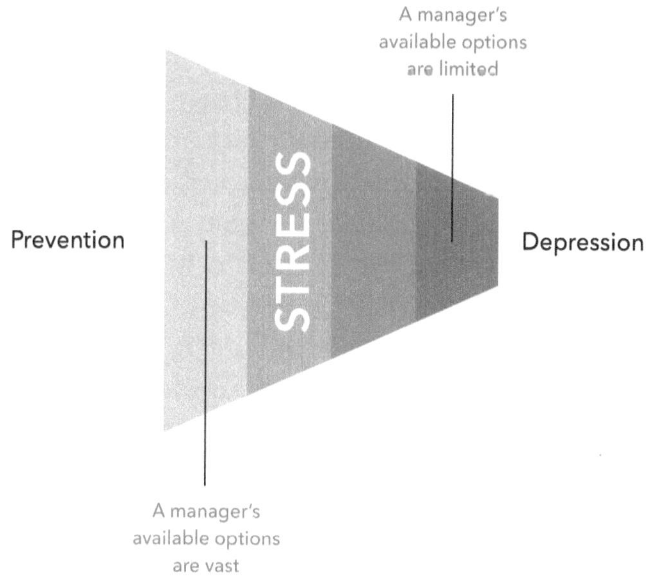

The employee's responsibility

We often hear stressed employees say, "My manager didn't do anything to prevent it. She should have been able to see how badly I was doing . . ." But a manager can't read an employee's thoughts. A manager can't look into their employees and know how they are doing.

If, as a manager, you are to have the possibility of intervening in time and helping an employee reach a solution, then you need to be made aware that there is a problem. When an employee suddenly breaks down and says "it's all too much", it would have made a huge difference if the employee in question had considered themselves earlier and thought: "I don't feel like I usually do. I'm reacting differently. I've a short fuse. I'm feeling under pressure. What caused it? And what can help me get well again?"

But it can be difficult or impossible for an employee to make that analysis by themselves if they have already reached the stage where they want to storm into your office and say that it has all become too much. It's the very nature of stress that by that point, they can't help themselves – because they are experiencing irrational and negative thoughts about themselves. So it's far more important that together we practise regularly talking about the experience of pressure as soon as we notice its onset.

Stress prevention is primarily about insisting on a dialogue and about how we can make a plan together once the first symptoms appear. For managers to be able to help find a solution, it requires mutual trust between them and the employee, and a safe work environment.

This brings us to an important point in relation to stress prevention management: much of the stress prevention work for which you are responsible can't really be done when things are about to fall apart and an employee is experiencing symptoms of stress. It has to be done in what you could call *peace time*. It's in peace time – when there are no pressing difficult cases, but peace and stability in the employee group – that, as a manager, you have to share how you would like to work together to handle symptoms of stress if they occur. It's also in peace time that you have to tell your employees what they can expect of you and what you expect of them. And it's in peace time that you have to talk to your employees about how stress prevention is a shared responsibility, about the importance of mutual openness if you are to be able to help, and about the communication between colleagues and the necessary follow-up.

As humans, we are all responsible for finding out what we need. We need to ask for help when it comes to whatever we ourselves can't find a solution to. This applies regardless of whether you are a manager or an employee. Your employees have a responsibility to go to you if they are experiencing pressure – even if that pressure isn't due to work. They should involve you and help you by telling you what they need. Or by telling you that they need management, leadership and support. But once you know that it can be difficult for an employee to share these things with you directly, then you can practise meeting your employees halfway, so that symptoms of stress don't develop.

The 4 Steps

Now that we have been through the introduction, it's time to get started with the four parts of the book, which together form the stress prevention management method. The four steps in stress prevention management are:

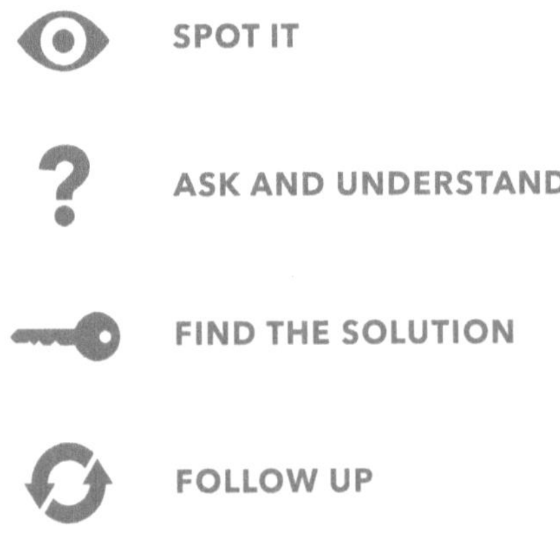

SPOT IT

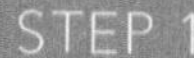

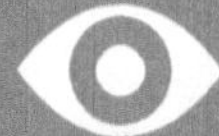

Stress starts with small changes.

Be aware if your employee
is reacting differently to usual.

Keep an eye out for behavioural changes.

DETECT CHANGES EARLY ON

If you notice an employee changing, it may be a good idea to give them more attention to find out if they are indeed developing stress. Pay attention to how they act in different situations. Do they seem openly pressured? Have they begun snapping at others, or are they complaining every day about the food being served in the canteen? Sometimes you can see clear signs that something isn't as it should be. At other times, you have to look behind the façade to detect whether what the employee is complaining about is actually a cover-up for the onset of stress.

Early signs of stress and the symptoms of stress may differ widely, as we've already mentioned, and this will often be difficult for you to spot because it's something the employee is struggling with and would rather not talk about. So listed below is an overview of such signs to make it easier for you. This will help you get to know what your employee is experiencing and what you can urge your employees to be aware of in themselves.

Early signs of stress

PHYSICAL SIGNS OF STRESS
(felt by the employee)
- Headache
- Dizziness
- Feeling uneasy in their body
- Palpitations
- Muscular tension
- A tendency to sweat
- Shortness of breath
- Dry mouth
- Infections
- Stomach pain
- Frequent desire to urinate
- Changes in the appetite
- Nausea
- Constipation
- Diarrhoea
- Reduced sex drive

MENTAL SIGNS OF STRESS
(felt by the employee)
- Excessive thoughts
- Negative, self-criticising or reproachful thoughts
- Worry
- Anxiety
- Mood swings, feeling depressed
- Shame
- Feeling to blame, having a guilty conscience
- Irritability, anger

- Tiredness
- Problems sleeping
- Difficulty remembering and concentrating
- Indecision
- Low self-confidence
- Cries easily

These symptoms are normal reactions and the majority of people are familiar with them. You're probably even familiar with them yourself. But even if you recognise many of the symptoms, it doesn't necessarily mean you need to be concerned. However, if you notice changes such as those listed above in one of your employees – or in yourself – over a number of weeks, there may be good reason to pay particular attention. Because problems don't occur when you respond to something you have noticed, but rather when you don't react to the change or perhaps even get used to it. Take action while you can. If an employee tells you or indicates that they have had a headache or pain in their stomach over a long period, then you should investigate what is behind the reaction.

The negative thoughts and feelings of an employee who is feeling under pressure often contribute to the employee not seeking help from either you or others. The changes often come about subtly and gradually. Perhaps they don't even realise that things are developing in a negative direction. They may think that they just need to pull themselves together or that seeking help won't make a difference anyway. They may be feeling ashamed, which, in turn, impedes them from telling others how they are doing. They may, justly or not, have thoughts of being subjected to unreasonable pressure from you. Therefore, you often won't be told about how they are doing.

The previous two lists cover the invisible signs of stress. But as we have seen, you can't expect to receive information from your employee. So what are you supposed to do? It's likely there are also a number of visible changes that will be a little easier for you to spot. Initially, they may be small, imperceptible changes, but they could be signs of underlying stress and, therefore, it's important to notice them. Here is a list of the most common behavioural changes. In Step 2, we examine what you can do when you see these changes in an employee.

BEHAVIOURAL CHANGES
(visible to you as a manager)
- Lack of perspective
- Indecision
- Reduced enthusiasm and interest
- Avoidance behaviour
- Withdrawing socially
- Displacement activity
- Tension
- Cynicism and a lack of empathy
- Deteriorating hygiene
- Messy clothing
- Increased use of stimulants, such as coffee, sugar, nicotine and/or alcohol.

Now we're going to meet Lisa. With the help of her story, we illustrate what happens when an employee changes their behaviour, and what you as a manager need to be aware of.

Being overbooked and a duvet day

At an office in Aarhus, Lisa puts her head in her hands. What has she got herself into? She's just succeeded in selling three workshops to one of their biggest customers. Lisa can hardly believe it. The top managers are delighted. She should be happy, but suddenly she feels as if everything is crashing down around her. Because there's a problem. Her son turns 10 on the day of the first workshop, and her daughter is going to the national school football championships on the day of the second workshop. Lisa has promised to be there for her children. She rubs her temples, thinking "*How can I cope?*"

On her way to the canteen, she meets her manager, Jane. Jane smiles when she sees Lisa, but Lisa doesn't respond.

"What's up with you today?" Jane asks, elbowing her playfully as they stand beside each other in the queue in the canteen.

"Nothing!" Lisa exclaims annoyed.

"I was only asking. Has something happened?"

"No!"

They're quiet for a moment. Lisa looks up at the board with the day's specials.

"Vegetable lasagne, ugh."

They eat in silence, and Lisa quickly returns to her office, her thoughts ruminating on the three workshops. What should she do? Her thoughts are swirling, but she can't think of any answer. Then the trainee, Sarah, asks about the printer yet again, making Lisa so annoyed that she reacts by shouting. Sarah looks scared. Lisa slams her door and sits down behind her desk. She has to get this situation under control now. What will the customer say when she cancels? And what will her boss say? Not Jane, but the company's managing director. What if the customer is so dissatisfied that they close their account? Would she be fired? What Lisa most wants is to turn off the computer and go home. She doesn't usually feel like this. She's a middle manager and is accustomed to juggling many balls at the same time. She can handle pressure. Occasionally, she even thinks she actually enjoys it. She's often heard herself tell other people how it gives an edge to her job and makes her go the extra mile. She finds the experience of something being at stake thrilling. Except for now. Right now, everything is tumbling down around her.

Just then there's a knock on the door.

"Yes!" snaps Lisa.

Jane opens the door.

"Do you have a moment?"

"No!"

Jane goes into her office anyway.

"Sarah is standing by the printer, sniffling. What's wrong?"

Lisa sighs and points to a chair. Jane sits down. Then Lisa tells her about her dilemma.

"I think you should contact the customer and explain," says Jane, when Lisa has finished telling her about her predicament with the workshops, her son's birthday and her daughter's football championship.

"Explain?"

Lisa looks like someone who has just received terrible news.

"Yes. Listen, try to move the workshops, maybe you can find other dates," Jane continues.

"But what if they're not happy with that? What if . . ."

"Because of this? I think it'd take more than this!"

Lisa starts sweating, and is still annoyed, but does as Jane says: she sends an email to the client suggesting some other dates.

The next morning, Lisa wakes up early and checks her phone. No answer yet. She takes a shower and makes coffee. Still no answer. Then she drives to work. The traffic is already building up. Her thoughts revolve around only one thing: should she ring the customer? No, she tells herself. It's still early. They need to have a chance to see the email. But what if they're angry? Her thoughts race ahead much faster than the traffic. Lisa considers turning around. And is that the flu she can feel coming on too? Maybe she should just take a sick day to forget all about it and get back on her feet again. Just one day.

Just then the phone rings. It's Jane.

"Hi," exclaims Lisa, surprised.

"I just wanted to hear how it's going."

"Oh, thanks. Well . . . Um, not so good. I'm actually on the way into work, but I'm thinking about turning around. I'm not feeling great . . . I think maybe it'd better if I work from home today."

"Are you sick?"

"No . . . I don't know. The customer hasn't answered. It's such a mess, and I don't feel well."

"Come in to the office. Just for a couple of hours. I've a case I'd like you to look at. Just a quick look."

Lisa sighs.

"Okay."

At 10.30, they're finished with Jane's case. It wasn't particularly complicated, and Lisa wonders why Jane even asked for her help.

But now that she's here anyway, she might as well stay. She can always take a duvet day tomorrow.

The next day is the same. Lisa doesn't feel great and has actually decided to stay at home when a colleague calls. They aren't very close. But now the colleague suddenly needs Lisa's help.

"What are you up to?" Lisa asks, sitting at the lunch table with her arms crossed, staring at Jane.

"What do you mean?" asks Jane.

"Do you think I don't know what you're doing? That you rang to get me in here? And now you're getting other people to do it, too."

Jane takes a sip of water.

"You moping around at home, sad and lonely, doesn't help anybody. We need you here."

"I'm not sad! Or lonely. Thanks very much!"

"Ring the client now. Get it over and done with."

Lisa shakes her head, goes up to the buffet and serves herself a portion of the dish of the day. Maybe Jane is right. Maybe she should just get it over and done with.

Back in the office, she dials the customer's number with sweaty hands. She hardly dares breathe when they finally pick up.

"Yes, we've seen your email," says the friendly secretary on the phone. "And of course it's perfectly okay to change the dates this far ahead. We're just looking at what new dates suit us best."

Lisa breathes a sigh of relief. Was that all it took?

Is Lisa stressed?

Lisa responds with symptoms of stress and her behaviour has changed. Her reaction is by no means unusual, but as a manager you'll probably quickly notice that something is wrong. Lisa works hard, but apparently isn't overburdened with things to do. It doesn't seem as if the piles of papers on her desk are pressurising her. In fact, we don't hear much about the amount of work she has to do. Actually, we hear more about how much she loves her job. Yet we are in no doubt about her feeling under pressure. You can clearly sense it in the way she snaps at people and can't focus on anything. And when she's in her car on her way to work and is considering turning around, we know without doubt that she is feeling pressurised. But is she stressed?

In "the three-part model", which we showed on page 26, we explained how we typically react with symptoms of stress when we experience being under pressure: we ascertain that there is a strain. We experience and interpret the burden. And then we react to the experience. We all act the same way here, regardless of our gender, age or position. We respond in the same way when we perceive something as dangerous. But what we experience as dangerous and how much we can bear before we develop symptoms of stress is very different from person to person. And the symptoms of the reaction vary individually, too.

It's important when looking for the onset of stress that you remember symptoms vary from person to person. To find out what is going on with the employee facing you, you need professional curiosity.

Let's put Lisa into "the three-part model" to see the connection between *strain* → *experience* → *reaction.*

- **Strain**

  Lisa is to hold three workshops for the customer her managers most want to collaborate with. But she is unable to attend two of them, and now she finds herself in a predicament. What should she cancel – her plans with her children or work? So it's not the assignment itself – the three workshops – that are a burden for Lisa. The burden is the dilemma of the two workshops coinciding with events in her private life, which are important to Lisa.

- **Experience**

  The project itself is actually positive. Lisa feels that she's in demand, but because it coincides with private arrangements, she feels under pressure and the situation seems problematic to her. Lisa is afraid that whatever she chooses she will be letting someone down. It's a difficult situation for her, and she is immediately plagued by worries: what if she gets fired? What if her children are upset? Her thoughts begin to swirl in an irrational and negative direction, and she interprets the situation as being really serious. Much worse than those around her believe it to be. Jane tells her it's not that bad. But it is for Lisa. Her feelings (fear and worry) and interpretation ("I'll be letting down either the company or my children") is Lisa's experience of the strain.

- **Reaction**

  Lisa responds as if she were facing a major threat. She has a short fuse, she snaps at her colleagues and has difficulty concentrating. She can't cope with things. She withdraws socially at work and believes it's best if she stays home until she gets better. Lisa's reaction shows classic early signs of stress.

Acknowledge the experience

We *interpret* and *tackle* situations quite differently. Something you think is problematic may be experienced by someone else as quite straightforward. Some people feel pressure due to a delayed flight, because they don't know when the next flight is leaving. Others experience pressure when their diary is too full, because how are they supposed to have time to drop off and collect their children? For others again, the idea of a big presentation at work can cause them to go off course – what if they say something wrong?

The ways we react when we experience being under pressure have many common traits, but early stress reactions are always rooted in our individual interpretations. We can experience the same situation very differently and, therefore, we also react quite differently to it. Maybe, as you were reading about Lisa, you thought *"Really? It's only three workshops"*, but that isn't how Lisa experiences it. She is afraid of being fired, despite there being no external indication of such a reaction. Her boss hasn't said anything. The customer hasn't said anything. And Lisa's children haven't commented either. In fact, they are completely unaware of the situation. The scenarios are solely the product of Lisa's imagination. Although she usually copes with having a lot of things on her plate, she is now practically in overdrive. With every hour that goes by, her irrational thoughts take over more and more. The onset of stress is characterised by developing an increasingly irrational way of seeing a situation. And this often happens when we are left alone to ruminate on our thoughts.

What you, as a manager, think of the situation, whether you can *understand* your employee's thoughts and feelings, and whether you think the situation is a pressurised one, is really immaterial. Your employee's experience of pressure isn't up for discussion. When your employee experiences pressure, then that's how it is. But you can ask and talk to your employee about the interpretation that has led to their reaction, and help them solve the problem that way. Managers who are able to accept this premise can increase wellbeing and job satisfaction and prevent stress among their employees. So be quick to notice behavioural changes and be sincerely interested in how your employee is experiencing a situation.

WHEN SHOULD YOU BE WORRIED?

As we have said earlier, you can't count on an employee coming to you of their own accord and telling you they are showing early symptoms of stress. In addition to the lists on pages 42 and 44, you also need to be aware of whether an employee:

- Has difficulty adapting

- Is showing resistance

- Seems unsatisfied or negative

- Is avoiding taking on assignments

- Is pushing themselves unnecessarily

- Is acting inappropriately in social situations

- Is losing themselves in details rather than looking at the bigger picture

Negative thoughts

Although Lisa's reaction is quite normal, it isn't completely harmless. Lisa's experience and stress response can actually be harmful. Lisa quickly drives herself into a negative mind-set, which only amplifies her responses. This is a typical development in a stressful situation. This is why you should identify the symptoms and address them as early as possible – to avoid those signs being the first step in the development of more severe stress.

One of Lisa's symptoms is irritation: she is annoyed at Jane's "hi", at the lasagne in the canteen, and at the trainee's questions about the printer. She even ends up giving her a hurtful response. But Lisa's real problem is neither the lasagne nor the trainee. She would most likely also have been annoyed had the dish of the day been spring rolls. Something else is behind Lisa's reactions. Behind the snapping and hostile façade, Lisa is filled with negative thoughts and emotions: she's afraid of not being good enough. Afraid of failing. And she is afraid of disappointing her bosses and her children. Her thoughts about herself are undoubtedly negative too. She tries to withdraw socially, first behind a closed door at work and then by staying at home, perhaps in order to protect herself. Such a negative development will at some point cause an employee to pass the threshold of taking sick leave.

Isolation can typically be seen as a precursor to absence due to sickness.

In the figure "The Evil Cycle of Stress" you can see how Lisa's thoughts go round in circles, amplifying the symptoms.

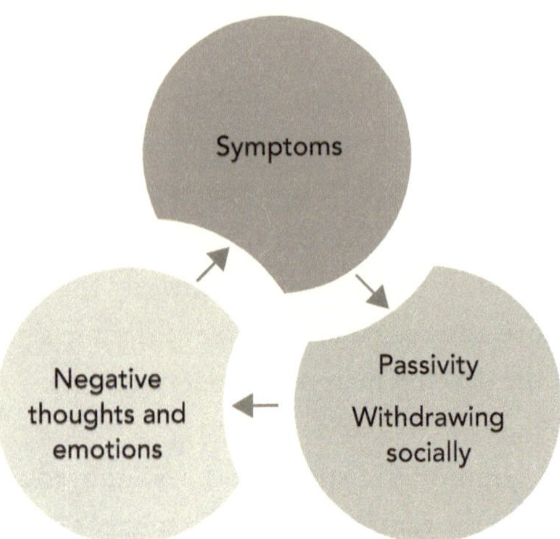

The Evil Cycle of Stress

Lisa fears what others will think of her – her boss, her colleagues and her children. In the aftermath of that fear, the idea of not being good enough comes with a feeling of guilt over ending up in the situation. The guilt weighs on Lisa. She's afraid both of being fired and of hurting her children. And she is ashamed of that. These are classic feelings that occur in everyone, when we experience symptoms of stress. Emotions are ancient and are linked to humankind's fear of exclusion from the community.

Four emotions that often occur with stress:

- Fear of the consequences; for example, fear of being fired. And of other people getting angry or upset with us.
- Feeling guilty about being unable to cope with what we think will happen.

- Shame at being unable to live up to our own or others' expectations of being a good parent, colleague or employee. This is almost equal to not being liked and no longer being a part of the flock.
- Sadness – accompanied by negative and worried thoughts about the past, present and future.

Difficult feelings and thought patterns interact with and affect each other. Here is a list of the thoughts experienced by most people as part of the early signs of stress when they are entering a negative spiral of irrational thoughts. When we show the list to those suffering from stress, they often nod and say, "That's exactly what I think". And as you can see, many of them are reflected in Lisa. Maybe you recognise them in some of your employees – or you yourself, too?

Typical thoughts

- Do my colleagues still like me?
- Is my boss upset with me?
- Am I going to be fired?
- How can I keep going like this?
- Am I good enough?
- My head can't take anymore . . . When I turn on the computer, I get dizzy and feel unwell.
- I forget things.
- Will I ever get back to my usual self?
- Maybe I'm just not cut out for this job. Or for any job.
- All my colleagues can do it, so why can't I?
- What is wrong with me?

- What must other people think of me?
- I can't cope with anything.

The irrational brain

The human brain has evolved over time so it's better able to analyse a problem and achieve a better result. This is extremely smart. It's how we improve, develop and manage to solve complicated problems. But it has a downside: if we experience being under pressure, that same analysis tool will always make us compare the state of things to something that is better and often ideal. This means that our thoughts will often negatively interpret the situation we are facing in any given moment. And one negative thought quickly leads to another negative thought. If we experience being under pressure, our thoughts will automatically head in a negative direction, which, in turn, brings up negative emotions and physical symptoms. Getting your thoughts back onto a more positive track may require some intervention. This is what Step 2 is all about.

SPOT IT - IN SHORT

- It begins with you as a manager. You must spot changes in your employees – you can't be sure your employees can do it themselves.
- Keep an eye on all kinds of changes; developing stress can manifest as both quite visible and almost invisible, subtle signs in an employee.
- Stress makes it harder to think rationally and talk about what is difficult, and stress also makes it more difficult to ask for help. The longer it takes you to intervene, the harder it will be to make a difference to the employee who is developing stress. And conversely, it's typically easier to achieve a common understanding and move in the right direction if you tackle the problem early on.
- The irrational-suffering-from-stress brain needs *management* and *leadership*. Your employee needs a manager: you. Open your eyes to everything happening around you so you can pick up on any early signs of stress.

If an employee comes to you about a colleague possibly being
stressed, you need to listen to them. If you are in any doubt
about the matter, it may be a good idea to observe the employee
for a short period of time – perhaps 1-2 weeks – while you try to
notice whether the employee in question is actually demonstrat-
ing some of the behavioural changes mentioned in Step 1.

If you are in doubt, it's also often a good idea to talk to the
employee you are concerned about and ask them how they are
doing. At times it will turn out they are fine, and then you have
erred on the side of safety. Remember that very few employees
will be annoyed at their manager asking them how things are
going for them, regardless of whether or not there's something
to worry about.

You can't always prevent the direction in which an employee
is heading – at least, not without them becoming aware of the
problem themselves. But you can talk openly about your concerns and make it clear to them that you expect them to take responsibility for their situation and their work, regardless of their
decisions. This way, you make the employee aware that they need
to be conscious of the risk of a negative development and the
consequences it may have. It shouldn't sound like a threat. But
you may need to mention it if the employee's work is affected,
and make it clear that, as a manager, you have to both help the

individual employee and do the best for the entire organisation. There may be a need for several conversations.

When it comes down to it, an employee knows best how they are doing. If they deny your observations, you can't force them to acknowledge them or agree with you. Talk openly with your employee about your concerns and make it clear that you expect them to take joint responsibility for their situation. Get involved as quickly as possible if there are assignments you need to address together. By doing this, you make them aware that they need to be conscious of both their reactions and behaviour. Sometimes, this is all it takes for the employee to get themselves back on track again. At other times it means you getting involved again at a later date, but by then the dialogue will already have begun.

If you have an employee who is completely unaware that something is wrong, several conversations will often be necessary. Here, it may also be necessary to include some reflections on the person's way of working, where you say something like, "I respect that you feel you aren't well. But I have to tell you that your way of working has changed, and, as a manager, I have to be aware of that too."

Monitoring is good, but it's important that the employees are aware of the goal behind it and experience it as a supportive measure and not as a form of control and pressure. Because that in itself can lead to stress. And the employee being contacted by someone who has no connection to the workplace and who may not even be in contact with the employee's manager isn't optimal either. The first person to contact an employee who is showing reduced wellbeing should be someone from inside the organisation, ideally the employee's immediate manager. It is the manager who has the possibility of making practical changes at work.

We are sceptical of the general spread of tests that don't actually lead to either a dialogue between the manager and the employee or to the curiosity and sincere interest that are needed to understand the employee's experience.

ASK AND UNDERSTAND

?

Start with an open conversation about what
is putting pressure on your employee.

Set aside your own interpretation for a while.

Tell your employee what you have observed.

Ask directly about your employee's
experience and interpretation.

Try to understand your employee's
experience of the situation.

Be clear about your intentions.

BE PROFESSIONALLY CURIOUS

We can't avoid stress and all of its complications by asking our employees to stop feeling, thinking and reacting. And we mustn't confuse stress prevention management with eliminating difficult or negative emotions in the workplace. Our emotions are precisely what make us whole as a person, someone who reacts when something isn't as we think it should be. Those reactions, which we addressed in Step 1 and call "early signs of stress" are, therefore, both natural and human. But, at the same time, they are precursors to or signs of mental health issues. The trick is learning to live with the reactions so they don't end up controlling us.

Here, in Step 2, we focus on *how* you, as a manager, help an employee from getting too deep into a vicious cycle of unpleasant feelings and thoughts and inappropriate reactions. We elaborate on what we mean when we say that you should "ask and understand" if you observe early signs of stress in an employee.

Avoidance behaviour impedes us

Stress prevention management is, to a high degree, about courage. As a manager, you should dare to ask what is going on when an employee responds unusually or inappropriately, even though it may feel uncomfortable and like you are crossing a boundary with them; you may feel like you are snooping into something that is private and doesn't concern you. Many managers are reluctant to talk to their employees about stress if they think it stems from something in their personal life. But stress at home affects the workplace too, and, as we wrote in the introduction, you should handle this in the same way as work-related stress. In fact, in most cases, stress is triggered by both private and work-related strain. Therefore, it makes no sense to distinguish between stress at home and work-related stress.

There is a natural reason why you and many other managers think it's wrong to interfere in something that may seem to be a private matter for the individual employee. When humans live in a natural environment, our survival depends on how good we are at avoiding risky and dangerous situations. Our brains still function like this, despite us being civilised. When we experience something as dangerous, our immediate reaction is still to avoid and flee because as humans, we are acutely encoded to believe that is the safest option. This is called avoidance behaviour. It is avoidance behaviour that controls us at work when we decide to "wait and see" instead of intervening, whether this relates to us experiencing the pressure ourselves or someone else around us experiencing it. Our brain perceives the situation as dangerous or unpleasant at the very least, and therefore we avoid it. There are important common traits in the mechanisms of an employee developing stress and a manager avoiding talking to the employee about it.

As a manager you probably avoid some of these difficulties because:

- You don't want to be friends with your employees.
- You're afraid of the answers you'll get if you ask what is wrong.
- You're nervous that what the employee is struggling with is too personal.
- You think everyone will get stressed if you use the word "stress" too much.

If we want to interrupt the stress curve, it's necessary to get something straight: **stress doesn't disappear by us not making it visible, hoping for the best and putting a lid on it**. So we have to break away from our avoidance behaviour, despite it being deeply engrained in each of us.

Tackle it today

Both you and your employee need to make an effort, and probably also to push the limits within yourselves to prevent the vicious cycle of negative emotions, thoughts and physical symptoms from ending in sick leave.

Your job as a manager is to be aware of whether an employee's behaviour is changing (see the list of "behavioural changes" in Step 1). Stick to the fact that you have noticed a change and that you would like to help – it's in the interest of the employee, the company and you as a manager. It isn't forbidden to ask an employee how they are. On the contrary, showing such interest can have a crucial effect.

Don't shy away from acting when an employee's manner changes. Don't wait until tomorrow; start asking the employee how they are doing today and be aware of how to do so. Some managers will intervene by writing an email. For a long time now, we have been dealing what is difficult via email, because there we don't have to be confronted with what we don't like in the same way as if we were to ring our employee or sit across a desk from them. But even though it's more convenient for us, this isn't the way to go. When we send emails back and forth in these situations, we run the risk of enlarging the gap between ourselves and our employee. And we are also very likely to start picturing each other as the enemy. You may think the employee should pull themselves together, be a little more positive and get on with their work. The employee might be thinking they're not right for the job at all, because you are expecting far too much of them. It could just boil down to a few private arrangements not fitting into their diary, like we saw in Lisa's case. It's difficult to be professionally curious via email, so it's necessary to talk face-to-face to each other so as to avoid such misunderstandings.

From avoidance to questions

Professional curiosity is the opposite of avoidance behaviour. When you are professionally curious, you show your employee that you care about them. You ask them often and directly how things are going for them. You listen to the answer without judging or commenting. If the employee experiences something as good or bad, then that's how it is for them. And whether or not you are of the same opinion, you recognise and respect this. When you are professionally curious, you put your own feelings aside – both the positive and the negative ones. When you are professionally curious, your goal is always to uncover the differences in the experience and interpretation of the situation, so as to then help the employee find realistic practical solutions that take them away from the experience of pressure and back to the experience of control.

That is exactly what Lisa's manager does in Step 1. Because what Lisa wants most of all is to escape from what feels difficult and stay away from work, Jane rings her. Jane has already expressed her opinion, but she can see that Lisa is still affected and recognises her experience of the problem. She doesn't say she's sorry for Lisa. Neither does she downplay the problem with comments such as "it'll be all right" or "it's nothing to get worked up over". She doesn't withdraw, despite no doubt wanting to. As a manager, Jane is curious about what she is observing: an employee whose behaviour has changed.

Professional curiosity
↓
Your understanding
↓
Communicate with the employee
↓
Shared understanding

Two crucial questions

Urging you to "ask and understand" is about you, as a manager, using your own observations as your starting point. In order to help an employee whose behaviour has changed, it's crucial that you familiarise yourself with what the employee is experiencing. Using professional curiosity, it's your job to find out two things:

- What is the employee experiencing, given that they are showing changes in their behaviour?
- How can you help the employee move away from the experience of pressure and back to an experience of control and wellbeing?

It's important for you to be aware that you don't need to take on board everything the employee is struggling with. Just because you invite an employee to have a conversation doesn't mean you now have to be friends with them and share everything that's going on in their life, and neither does it make you their therapist. But you need to have built a bridge between you and the employee so you understand when they are feeling under pressure, because the employee takes that feeling of being pressured with them to work no matter where it stems from, and it affects both the employee's work and how they are as a colleague. As a manager, it's about gaining knowledge of the employee's experience and response, which is necessary in order to help them in the right direction. This requires empathy, but you still need to have a professional relationship with them.

When we share our unpleasant thoughts and feelings with others, they often become less burdensome. Fewer negative thoughts and feelings equate to less anxiety and, thus, fewer symptoms of stress. And you don't need to push the boundary of either therapy or friendship when you ask an employee how they are doing, as long as you maintain your professional curiosity.

What you can say to an employee:

- I've noticed you haven't seemed very happy lately. Is that how you're feeling?
- I've noticed your work hasn't been up to its usual standard lately. And that you're avoiding taking on new assignments. Do you recognise this? What's your experience of the situation?

- It seems like something is going on. Your tone is different than usual – as if your fuse is shorter. Is there anything I should be aware of?

It's vital that you ask with genuine interest. You should be honest and concrete, without making the questions sound like an accusation. The employee has to see you and your interest as a helping hand; that you are interested in them and their wellbeing and would like to help find a solution.

When misunderstanding turns to conflict

A common occurring theme whenever employees and managers talk about stress is misunderstandings. Many periods of stress have started with a misunderstanding. Perhaps a situation arose which the manager and employee each interpreted in their own way and, therefore, reacted differently to. It could be changes in the workplace, such as colleagues being replaced or new work duties. The employee thought there was a problem and experienced unfairness, while the manager didn't view it as such. Each party was caught up in their own interpretation of the situation and in their emotions, which resulted in them being annoyed with each other.

That is what happened at the company you are going to discover now where a usually dedicated employee encountered unforeseen problems.

Dreams of working overseas

Peter's story

Peter lives and works in Copenhagen. The company he works for has grown in recent years. Several branches have been opened around the country, and many more employees have been taken on. Now they would like to expand abroad, and Peter's very interested in such a position. Management therefore offers him a job in the UK, where the first branch outside of Denmark is being established. Peter is thrilled. He can finally get started on the international career he's been dreaming of. And management is delighted to have a trusted member of staff as the first permanent employee in the new overseas branch. It seems to be a win-win solution.

Peter gets a nice office with a fine conference room for inviting new customers and business partners. Management also arranges a company car for him, just like he is used to at the head office. Peter moves to the UK and everyone is optimistic. But two months later, problems crop up.

Peter flies to Denmark to attend joint status meetings, which are held once a month. But he often looks sceptical at the meetings as he sits with his arms crossed. He seldom says anything. He used to be the one who chatted and smiled when everyone was together. If he says anything now, it's always negative and goes against management. Whether it's about the IT system, the Christmas party or customer contracts, Peter disagrees. Management doesn't understand at all. He got his international chance, just like he dreamed of, so what's the problem?

"I'm feeling under pressure," replies Peter, one day after the monthly joint meeting, when his immediate manager calls him into his office and asks what's wrong.

"Pressure?" asks the manager puzzled. "Over what?"

"Bookings, meetings, customers . . . There's too much to do, and I'm the only one doing everything over there."

The manager nods. Yes, Peter is all alone in the job in the UK, but it's only until they get one or two more employees. It takes time to find the right skills. And local demand needs to keep up too. They talked about all of this when they made the UK agreement. *How can this be coming as a surprise to him?* she thinks.

"I can't take on any more before Christmas," says Peter.

"But it's more than two months until then," his manager replies in amazement.

"Then you'll have to hire another person. I can't do any more than I already am!"

The manager nods again. If that's how Peter is experiencing the situation, they need to act accordingly. The manager promises Peter that she will talk to the rest of the management team about the overbooking he is experiencing so they can find a solution.

Once Peter has left the office, his manager looks at Peter' diary. All employees have access to each other's diaries. But when the overview appears on screen, his manager is surprised. There are four bookings a week in Peter' diary. Four! That's how many Peter used to have a day when he worked in Copenhagen. His manager starts wondering what's going on as she feels the irritation beginning to bubble.

If you were Peter's manager

Misunderstandings over diaries are classic. Perhaps you recognise this from your own everyday life: an employee experiences one thing and you experience something completely different. What would you do if you were Peter's manager?

1) Wait to see if it's just a phase Peter is going through – one that will pass?
2) Rely on your own judgement, be direct and ask him to pull himself together?
3) Ask Peter where the pressure he is experiencing is coming from – whether there is something besides the bookings that is burdening him?

We call this challenge "the manager's crossroads". It's a challenge that many managers face every single day. The figure illustrates your three options:

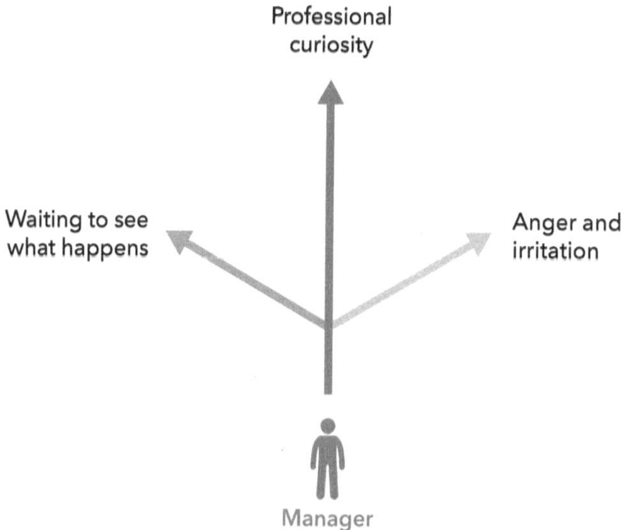

- **Option 1**

  You wait and see what happens. Of course, Peter's diary isn't full for the next two months; and, of course, he can take on more than he is doing now. Perhaps he is being pressurised by something at home, and you'll give him the opportunity to deal with that before you do anything else. You know Peter to be a skilled and loyal employee and you trust him.

- **Option 2**

  You have a conversation with Peter to clear the air, because his diary isn't full at all, so what is all this about? He knew the conditions before he left. You ask him to change his attitude. And to get back to work.

- **Option 3**

  You think there has to be something else going on. Peter says he's under pressure due to bookings, but you can see there aren't many of them in his diary. You set aside time to talk to Peter about how things are going. You are honest with your questions and curiously ask what is making him experience being under pressure.

Without thinking too much about it, many managers choose options 1 or 2. Either they wait or they say something negative to the employee. It's obvious that Peter isn't correct in his claim of being under pressure when you see that his diary isn't full, and you know he can manage much more. This is a reaction based on your own – in this case rational – assessment; he's actually not as busy as he says he is. But if you interpret and assess how Peter is feeling, the situation is likely to take a turn for the worse, which can easily lead to severe stress and absence due to sickness.

When things go awry

Imagine your thoughts are like a cog. When you collaborate with others and you perceive work in the same way, your individual cogs align with each other and work as they move in sync. But if we end up having different interpretations of the same situation, the cogs lose contact with each other, rotate in different directions or stall. You see things one way. Your employee perceives them in another. This can happen with changes, an increased workload and such like. In those situations, we can literally talk about "things going awry".

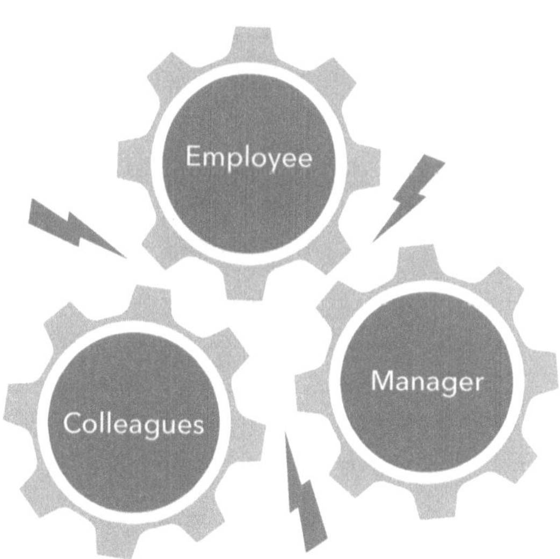

When the cogs aren't in contact with each other, it can lead to further misunderstandings and viewing each other as the enemy, which is what happens in Peter's story. The cogs have long since gone awry by the time Peter and his manager sit down to talk. His manager has begun viewing Peter as the enemy instead of as her helper. His manager believes that Peter's way of thinking isn't rational. But as we described in Step 1, the stressed brain is characterised precisely by being irrational. The manager's rational arguments, such as "I can't see any more than four bookings" or "In Copenhagen you were able to take many more than four" don't mean anything to Peter.

If you want to increase the wellbeing of your employees and reduce stress-related sick leave, you need to intervene early on, actually as soon as the employee is showing signs of being under pressure, and when you find yourself at the crossroads you need to choose option 3: look behind the employee's – and your own – immediate responses and enter into the brewing conflict with professional curiosity. This means that you step out of your normal, problem-solving-leadership role for a while and into a space of investigative curiosity. You don't react instinctively with irritation or try to rationally understand the employee, but rather take on the role of listener, where you try to understand the employee's own experience. This isn't necessarily the same thing as accepting it or agreeing with it, and it doesn't mean you forget about being a manager. We can say that with professional curiosity you are both a step ahead of the employee and a step behind them. You are at once aware that the employee's interpretation can be characterised by irrational thinking and openly interested in the employee's own way of seeing the situation.

Being present from a distance

Stress prevention management is about being present for each employee as an individual person. Maybe you work in a company where you are scattered across the country or there are a thousand kilometres between you and your employees, just as we saw in the example of Peter, who was all alone in the UK. You may, therefore, find it difficult to see how you're supposed to be able to notice behavioural changes. Indeed, paying attention to employees with whom you don't share a location undoubtedly demands something extra from you as a manager. But if you decide that this attention is a vital part of your management and leadership, then it doesn't have to be impossible.

When Peter moves to the UK, there are suddenly more than a thousand kilometres between him and his manager. This is where the cogs begin to lose contact with each other. Peter is obviously experiencing being in the UK differently from how management thinks he is experiencing it. Much has changed for Peter: new country, new city, new department, no colleagues . . . And he reacts to all of that. But management continues to view Peter as they usually do and as they view all the other employees. For them, there is no difference between Peter at the head office in Denmark and Peter in the UK. But there is for Peter. It takes some time before management becomes aware that there is a problem. His manager waits to see what happens before inviting Peter in to have a talk. The first joint meeting where Peter sat with his arms crossed could be about something entirely different. Perhaps he was just in disagreement with the specific topic being discussed at the meeting. Maybe he was busy or tired. While the manager waits, Peter's symptoms of stress worsen. As he still seems to be unlike his normal self at the third joint meeting, his manager begins to wonder about Peter's behaviour. Only then does she ask him in for a chat to hear about how things are going.

Because the manager has seen that Peter's diary isn't actually overbooked, as Peter himself thinks it is, his manager takes a few days to consider her response. The manager's immediate reaction is to get annoyed at Peter. But then she speaks to the rest of the management team, who agree that there must be something else going on given that Peter is responding as he is. Now they want to find out what is really going on. Peter's manager travels to the UK. From conversations and by following Peter up close, the manager realises what could be the real reason for Peter's frustrations. Even before lunch on the second day, she can feel her own thoughts changing and going off in a way that isn't rational. She gets frustrated with little things and lets details that normally wouldn't bother her get her down. She can see how lonely it is to be in the office all on your own. And loneliness is often the driving force for negative, irrational thoughts that lead to an experience of more loneliness. As they work together in the office over a few days, they gain a common understanding of Peter's experience of feeling isolated and being solely responsible for the work in the UK. When the manager travels back to Copenhagen two days later, she is happy. She is going to be with her other colleagues at the head office again, but, above all, she's happy because she and Peter have found a plausible reason for his change in behaviour. Along with the rest of the management team, she decides to no longer focus on the problem of the diary. It's not about whether there are too many or too few bookings, but about emotions and, in this case, the experience of being the only one doing all the work. Therefore, the manager is going to focus on solving that problem.

Peter's story can also be used to illustrate the isolation process and loneliness that occurs in most instances of stress. This also helps explain why stress is so prevalent among people who are unemployed.

As Peter's isolation becomes visible, his manager acts in a more stress-preventative way. In the weeks that follow, she rings Peter at least every other day. Most often, they only talk for five minutes, but a couple of times the conversation lasts up to 25 minutes. The manager thinks that's a long time and sometimes she feels she doesn't have time for it. But then she starts working out how much one-to-one attention her employees at head office get from her if they need it, and it turns out to be equal to what she is now using on Peter. In their frequent conversations, neither Peter nor his manager talk about emotions. They don't dwell on how Peter is doing. Peter doesn't get fewer assignments. Peter does, however, talk about his work and the cases he is dealing with. Which project is in focus now? Who is the contact person? What is going well? What is not going as expected? How can Peter improve on what isn't working optimally? What should Peter do for the rest of the day?

The result of the frequent contact is an employee who thrives. And Peter isn't going to be taking sick leave any time soon. A few months later, his diary has up to eight weekly bookings. Management has realised that when it comes to stress prevention, general employee benefits aren't enough. If a manager isn't aware of the individual employee's wellbeing, the cogs can go awry – the employee can begin isolating themselves. However, management now has what it takes to quickly rectify the situation whenever dissatisfaction, which could end in stress-related sick leave, occurs. They know that it requires an extra effort and that they must invest time in it. But they also know that it pays off.

Stay on the riverbank

You probably already know much of what we write about professional curiosity. And you may have even though *what's new here?* while you were reading. You already talk to your employees. But we suggest that it's difficult for you to practise professional curiosity. At least it is for many of the managers we have spoken to and for ourselves as managers. Professional curiosity is a management skill that needs to be developed and honed. One of the best ways of being good at working with it is to imagine yourself on a riverbank.

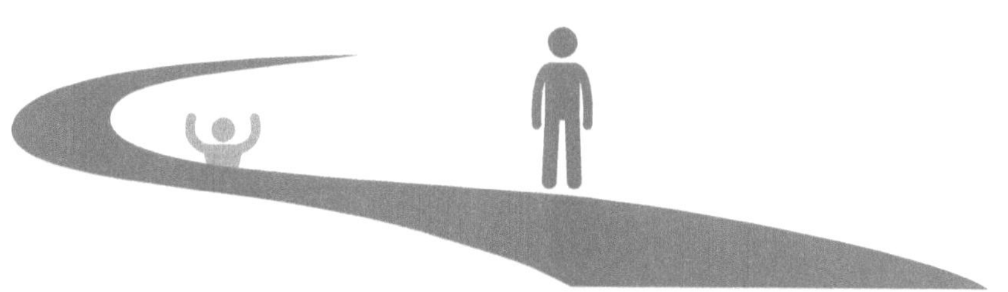

When, like Peter's manager, you become aware that the behaviour of one of your employees has changed and you intervene, it's crucial that you aren't being affected by your own feelings or opinions if you're going to succeed in stopping the stress. We've borrowed a concept that we call "staying on the riverbank", from *Acceptance and Commitment Therapy*, as it very nicely illustrates the situation that you often find yourself in as a manager when an employee ends up out of balance.

Imagine standing on the bank of a river. The employee is in the water. The river represents everything that is happening in the employee – thoughts, feelings, physical experiences. The current whirls them around; it's strong and increases every day as you watch it. Their experience is that they have lost control of their everyday life and can't reach the shore on their own. It's also difficult for them to navigate while they are in the river. They have difficulty seeing which bank is closest. They make irrational decisions. They may even swim in the wrong direction.

To help the employee, you must remain standing on the river-bank. Your employee needs your overview, your leadership and your management. It can be challenging to stay there. Your intuition tells you to jump into the river, and you're probably even getting "invitations" to do so. Perhaps the employee's behaviour evokes emotions in you – these could be compassion, irritation or other emotions. Feelings that tempt you to jump into the river without yourself being aware of it – this is your own intuitive reaction. The employee can have feelings, such as anger and fear – strong emotions that affect those close by. But if you do become affected by their feelings, you will immediately end up like your employee: a whirl of negative emotions and irrational thoughts. We often only see this first when we have already jumped from the bank and are in the river with the employee. And this can lead to reproach, distrust, pity, misunderstanding and much more.

Peter's manager is about to jump into the river when Peter says his diary is overbooked. His manager wants to react to that, but it would make her annoyed and angry, just like Peter already is. However, she chooses to remain standing on the bank and does everything possible to understand the problem rather than getting swept along by it.

Staying on the bank isn't the same as being indifferent to the employee. Being able to remain on the bank – or return to the bank if you've fallen into the river – is a crucial prerequisite for professional curiosity. When you are on the riverbank, you're able to get an overview of the situation and offer your employee your help as a manager. You are of almost no use to your employee if you are treading water down in the river with them. But if you stand on the bank, you can help find a solution that will bring your employee back to the bank and give them an experience of having control over their everyday life again.

ASK AND UNDERSTAND - IN SHORT

- Be curious.
- Be persistent – there may be a need for several conversations to uncover the employee's interpretation to reach a joint understanding.
- Focus on understanding first – and then on finding a solution – with the employee; in that way, you ensure that the solution makes sense to the employee.

I haven't had any training in having difficult conversations. So wouldn't it be better for me not to talk to an employee who seems to be going through a hard time?

A somewhat clumsy conversation is better than no conversation at all. More important than formal training in conversation skills and techniques is standing by your observations, describing them and being clear in your communication regarding the purpose of the conversation with the employee; emphasising that you want what's best for them.

What are you not allowed to ask about?

Professional curiosity means trying to gain knowledge about what is needed in order to help an employee work at their best and avoid getting sick. You need to be aware if you cross a boundary and touch too closely upon something. Don't go in for unlimited openness, and respect that there are things that the employee would prefer to keep to themselves. There may also be legal, cultural or company rules regarding what a manager can and can't ask an employee. And remember that managers must not ask employees questions regarding diagnoses.

Remember that you are a manager, not a psychologist or a doctor. You can't and shouldn't diagnose your employees. That said, you must react on the basis of your observations and share them with your employee. You can keep your reflections within your area and say, "I see that your manner has changed . . .", "it's quite possible you already have it under control, but if it were me, I think I'd . . ." or "I don't know if this is of any use to you, but my experience tells me . . ."

If you're very concerned about your employee, you need to be more insistent regarding seeking professional health care; for example, that they go to their doctor. For you, as a manager, it may be a question of them not being able to do their job satisfactorily enough if they don't get better. You may have to say this to emphasise the importance of them seeking help.

FIND THE SOLUTION

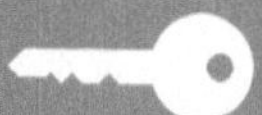

Help the employee regain control.
Pay attention to the employee's - and your
own - need to experience fairness.

Find out with your employee
what can actually help them, both
now and in the long term.

Be open to the employee's own
suggestions - and be ready to take
control if the employee doesn't have any.

ENABLE THE EMPLOYEE TO TAKE BACK CONTROL

As a manager, you've probably learned that listening to employees is important. Because by listening you are better able to handle conflicts. But being accommodating isn't enough when it comes to preventing stress. For the employee who is experiencing early symptoms of stress, being listened to and understood isn't enough. As a manager, you have to ensure that you reach a concrete solution that brings the employee away from the experience of stress and back to an experience of being in control of what is happening. If the employee can't reach a solution on their own, it's your job to help. And you do that by being more specific than you might think is necessary. We will return to this later.

Here in Step 3, we focus on two of the most important concepts in stress prevention management:

- Control
- Fairness

Let's start with control. In recent years, several studies have shown that the experience of control is crucial to human welfare. But before we take a closer look at these studies, you're going to meet an employee who experiences what it's like to lose control.

His two managers tackle the situation each in their own way. When you read the story, notice how their help affects Henry, the employee, in different ways.

Do the best you can

Henry's story

Henry works in a government department. He is ambitious and thorough. The type who sticks to his word and who often goes the extra mile. An employee that most managers dream of having in their department. But one Friday afternoon, Henry feels overwhelmed. There are a pile of tasks for him to do on his desk and he would like to do them all properly, but he realises that no matter what he does, he won't be able to finish them all by the agreed deadline. It's a problem. Henry knows that being late will affect the minister, other politicians and journalists, and that puts pressure on him. As does the thought of what other people must think. His colleagues, his bosses, everyone. What will the consequences be? He should have excused himself earlier; it's too late now. He is sweaty and has difficulty concentrating. When a colleague asks if Henry wants to go for lunch, he shakes his head and puts on his headphones. Lunch? He has absolutely no appetite.

Henry stands up an hour later. He feels dizzy and has to grab the edge of the desk to prevent himself falling over. When Henry recovers, he makes a decision. He goes to his head of office, John, and explains: he has said yes to too many things because they sounded exciting and because he wanted to make a good impression on his colleagues, but now things are slipping. He can't possibly get everything done within the timeframe. What should he do?

John answers: "I don't think there's much to do about it now. You'll just have to do the best you can."

"But," Henry objects, "what about all the things I won't be able to get done?"

"You'll have to do what's most important and leave the rest to next week."

"But it's all important! I don't know where to start."

"You'll have to prioritise – that's what we all have to do. You don't have to do everything 100 per cent," John replies, his body language signalling that the conversation is over.

Confused, Henry goes out into the corridor. Some of his colleagues are heading home.

"Have a nice weekend," they say.

Henry doesn't answer. With a stiff look, he goes to the kitchen to get a glass of water. When he comes out, he can't remember what he was going to do next.

"Hi Henry," he suddenly hears behind him.

Henry turns. Behind him is the head of department, Sally.

"Well, are you heading off for the weekend, too?" asks Sally.

"No," says Henry curtly. "I don't think there'll be any weekend for me."

"What? Has something happened?"

Henry looks down.

"There's just so much going on. And everything has to be finished now. I don't know how . . ."

"Come with me," Sally says, steering him towards her office.

Henry follows. Sally closes the door behind them.

"You don't usually say things like that. Is it something to do with work or is there something else going on?" asks Sally when they are sitting down.

Henry shakes his head. It's just work. But that's enough. He knows he bears the responsibility for the piles on his desk. No one asked him to take on so much, but he still feels like "the newbie", despite working at the ministry for almost a year. He feels a great need to show his colleagues that they can count on him. The problem is now he's going to end up showing the exact opposite: that he can't be counted on and that he's no good.

"I can hear that you're bogged down with work right now," says Sally. "What help do you most need to move forward?"

Henry thinks about it. "Right now everything is a mess and I honestly don't know what to do. I probably need some advice on how to deal with the situation here and now. And on how to get an overview of things, get some perspective."

"I think you have to write to the others and tell them that you've been delayed. It won't be the first time they'll have received an email like that. I'll clear it with John."

"But can I do that?" says Henry nervously. "What will they think?"

"It's annoying when someone delays another person's work, but they might find themselves in that boat one day. You can say that it's in agreement with John and me. And I'd suggest you draw up a list of what you need to get done, so that you get an overview of the tasks at hand. It's good to get things out of your head and down on paper. When you come in on Monday, come to me so we can talk about how you can prioritise all that needs to be done and how you can avoid having loads of simultaneous deadlines in the future. What do you think of that?"

Henry nods. That's exactly the advice he needs. He goes back to his desk and does as Sally has asked. Two hours later he goes home for the weekend – tired and hungry, but mostly relieved.

Control is the keyword

When you guide your employees, it's crucial that you do it in a way that gives the employees an experience of being in control. A Swedish PhD thesis recently established the importance of this for stress-related disorders (ref. 12).

The experience of control is one of the key phrases for wellbeing. Many employees who feel stressed and have symptoms of stress recognise the experience of not being in control. They feel they are stuck and unable to act. Some of the typical things they say include:

- "I can't take any more, but . . ."
- "I can't change it – that's how the job is."
- "At my age, it isn't possible to change jobs."
- "I can't get by without my salary."
- "My manager won't change – there's nothing I can do."
- "As a mother of young children, I just don't have enough time for everything."
- "In our industry, you are constantly on the move – otherwise you're out of the running."

If you're going to help one of your employees, you need to support them in finding and implementing a good solution for them that helps them experience control. However, there are two traps you need to be aware of.

The first trap is thinking that as the manager you have sole responsibility for solving the problem. That you have to find a solution that you think makes sense, without involving the employee.

This may solve the problem here and now, but it doesn't give the employee the experience of having strategies to handle any difficulties and take control of the situation. The employee will feel supported in the short term and will probably also appreciate the help, but the next time something is challenging, they will again have difficulty knowing what to do.

The second trap is leaving the employee to find a good solution on their own. The "with-freedom-comes-responsibility" management style can be appropriate in some contexts, but not when dealing with a stressed brain. As we have mentioned a few times, an employee who is experiencing pressure and is already showing stress responses is likely to be unable to find a solution themselves, because a brain in the early stages of stress has already entered an irrational and negative train of thought. There is neither perspective nor thoughtfulness here, but rather negative thoughts and feelings such as anxiety, guilt and shame. And those feelings affect our judgement. Employees, such as Henry, who are otherwise skilled and usually in control of their working day, can therefore be incapable of finding the solution themselves. When he is told that he has to prioritise the work himself, the negative thoughts and the feeling of inadequacy take hold even more, because that is precisely what he is having difficulty with. He has lost control.

But if, as a manager, you don't help the employee by solving the problem for them – and equally, you can't expect the employee to solve it themselves – then what concrete action can you take? The solution is found in the interaction between you and your employee. Just like Henry and Sally.

Help with getting an overview

Henry experiences pressure that almost pulls the rug out from under him in just a few hours. He reacts with symptoms of stress. But he makes a good decision when he goes to his manager and asks for help. The manager's answer, "You'll just have to do your best" and "you don't have to do everything 100 per cent" doesn't support Henry in the specific situation. The manager's intentions are good. He wants the best for Henry. And he believes he is helping by not pushing an employee in a difficult situation. The problem is, Henry isn't being helped back to a place of control. Instead, he is left with an even greater experience of feeling overwhelmeda nd having neither control nor the power to take action. He goes into the kitchen, but forgets what he was doing when he comes out again. Most people have done this at some point in their lives. Seen in isolation, it isn't dangerous. And neither is it dangerous if one day you aren't hungry enough for lunch or eat later because you have something that needs to be finished. But if a situation such as Henry's isn't addressed, the employee will head into a weekend of negative thoughts and a lot of worrying.

When Henry stops to think about it, he realises he's not feeling well – neither physically nor mentally. So how will he feel on Monday morning? Avoidance behaviour almost certainly comes into play here, too. Many employees will reach the conclusion that taking a sick day is the best solution, if the problem waiting for them feels huge or unmanageable, and they can't see a solution. A day at home can be quite appealing. Everyone knows stress is dangerous. Peace and quiet will definitely help. Won't it?

Fortunately, Sally helps Henry out of his negative thoughts. Sally notes that Henry isn't his usual self and she asks why. Based on a common understanding of the situation, together they find a practical solution that works.

OUT OF YOUR HEAD AND DOWN ON PAPER

- When we write things down instead of trying to remember everything at once, we get more of an overview of things.
- Help your employee get an overview by making lists of concrete tasks and responsibilities with them.
- Sort out and prioritise the employee's work together. The employee can often set priorities themselves, but they need you to approve the prioritisation.
- Use the lists in the future, so you both know when the employee has reached their goals and finished their work. And then follow up on the points on the lists.

Can a single experience, such as that of Henry's, really lead to a more serious stress condition? Yes, it can. A situation like that, where unpleasant thoughts and emotions begin to take hold, can be the first step to an employee losing track of things, feeling discomfort at the thought of work, experiencing pressure and being scared because they can't see how to regain control.

In this context, it's vital to be aware that you can actually reinforce negative, self-critical thinking and shame in the employee if all you do is reduce an employee's workload after they have told you they are under pressure. This can be perceived as "proof" by the employee that they're no good for anything and can't deliver what is expected of them. As we mentioned earlier, the right solution requires curiosity – sometimes a reduction in the workload is the right thing to do, but at other times something else entirely is needed.

Steering, support or development?

There are many ways to lead and manage. As a manager, you've probably been introduced to several models, all of which describe management from a particular angle. When it comes to stress prevention management, you can take a slightly different view of management and leadership. Here, it's about finding a way to lead that creates the best conditions for supporting and developing your employees, so that wellbeing can be created.

We often talk about two basic types of managers today:

- **The task-orientated manager,** who sets goals for the employee and delegates tasks.
- **The relationship-oriented manager,** who focuses on the employee's development and has a more supportive approach to management.

Several years ago, experts began to agree that the relationship-oriented manager has the most positive effect on employees. In 2004, researchers from the University of Florida came to the conclusion that if you focus more on development than on goals, your employees will thrive (ref. 13). And as recently as 2015, a Danish study showed that Danish managers are actually best at steering, while they struggle a little with inspiring and developing their employees (ref. 14).

The interesting thing is that Henry's manager, John, believes he is practising relationship management. He has convinced himself that he's supporting Henry by saying he should do his best. He has attended a course and learned that it's important to acknowledge his employees, and now he would like to show Henry it's okay that he is experiencing a difficult situation, but that as a manager he trusts him and won't put additional pressure on him.

As a starting point, it's considerate of the manager to signal to Henry that it's okay he can't get everything done. And that he is confident that Henry can prioritise his own work. But that's not actually what John says to Henry. He says he *should be able* to prioritise his own work. Thus, Henry's manager falls into the same trap that many managers subconsciously end up in, even if their intentions are good: the manager gives Henry full responsibility. He indirectly demands that Henry solves his own problem. But he gives him no tools for *how* to do so. And that makes the situation even worse for Henry. He *knows* that he should have control over his work. And he usually does. He is known as "the efficient one". The problem is, he is feeling overwhelmed and so the manager's well-meaning advice reinforces his looming sense of shame and insecurity.

The combination of great responsibility/high demands and no control/low influence is almost a direct path to discontent, dissatisfaction and symptoms of stress. In particular, research shows that this causes depressive symptoms. And this has been known since the 1970s, when the "demand-control model" that we described in the introduction was developed. The demand-control model emphasises that depressive symptoms are often the consequence when we discover we aren't in control and that we are simultaneously subject to great demands. What happens to Henry – his change of mood, lack of overview, forgetfulness, reduced appetite, sweating and dizziness – are symptoms indicating that he is experiencing pressure that he doesn't know how to deal with. He is usually in control, but despite his job requirements being the same, he experiences a loss of control.

HIGH DEMANDS = HIGH MENTAL DEMANDS

- Heavy workload

- Fast pace of work

- Pressed for time

- Complex assignments

LOW CONTROL

- Little influence on the planning and preparation of work

- Little influence on crucial decisions

- Poor opportunities for developing and using new skills; for example, doing very routine work or work that gives little opportunity for learning something new

HIGH DEMANDS + LOW CONTROL = RISK OF DEPRESSION

In 2017, the Danish National Research Centre for the Working Environment and a number of other research units from three other countries studied whether high demands and low control can also lead to depression that requires treatment (ref. 15). They investigated not only whether or not this combination brought about symptoms, but also whether it could make people sick.

And they discovered that it can. 14 studies involving a total of 120,000 subjects pointed to the same conclusion:

The experience of high demands and low control can lead to depression. The more often a person experiences high demands being placed on them, while simultaneously not having a high degree of control or influence, *the higher the risk of being admitted with depression. The result turned out to be valid regardless of gender, age, title and background.* So, apparently, it doesn't matter what type of organisation you work in or what type of management team you are part of. The experience of being in control is central for both you and your employees.

That's why control is so important

When we talk about the feeling of being in control, it isn't about having to control everything that happens in our lives. That is neither possible nor something we should strive for. There are many conditions that we can't change. But most people know the experience of taking control at important times. And it's precisely that feeling of being able to act and influence your life and situation that is vital – in many cases, more important than the conditions you have to accept.

When we know the experience of being able to act and affect our situation, we feel safe – even when it is difficult. It isn't dangerous *per se* to experience not being in control. Most people experience this occasionally. Adversity and difficulty are part of life, no matter what we do. The American psychologist Julian Rotter described this as early as in the 1950s. He introduced the world to the concept of "locus of control", which is still quite relevant today (ref. 16). "Locus of control" describes the difference between:

- The experience of having control – being able to greatly influence the things around you and experiencing that you influence what happens (left side of the figure).
- The experience of not being in control – things just happen without you controlling what happens, when it happens and how it happens (the right side of the figure).

Julian Rotter was concerned with investigating why some people are fundamentally influenced by the experience that control over what is happening to them lies predominantly outside them. This could be in the environment or in external circumstances (external locus of control). Conversely, other people are characterised by having an experience and belief that situations and results are due to their own personal capabilities and skills (internal locus of control).

Subsequent research has shown that people with an internal locus of control generally perform better when dealing with stress and disease than people with an external locus of control. If we let ourselves be inspired by Rotter's concepts, but think of them more as different ways to experience a situation, then depending on how you are doing, it can be illustrated as follows:

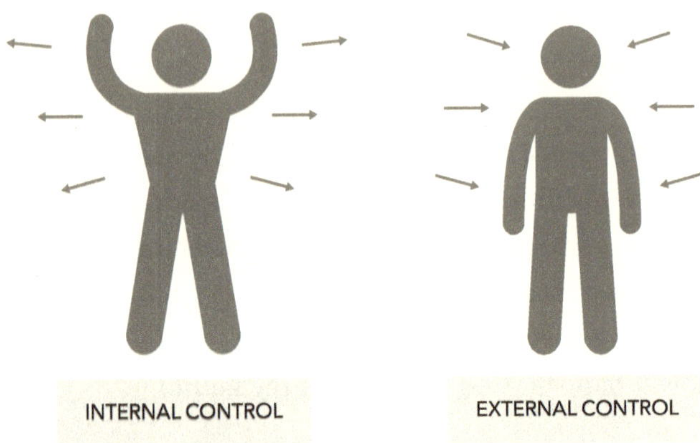

MODEL: Locus of control, inspired by Julian Rotter

Many managers find that the locus of control model makes sense when helping an employee with underlying symptoms of stress find concrete solutions. If one of your employees remains in a state of things "just happening" and the person becomes more and more incapable of action, you need to step in and help them move towards an experience of there being something they can contribute to influencing.

Sometimes the employee themselves can get to a place where they experience being able to influence their life and what is happening around them. At other times, they need help to move in the right direction. When you, as a manager, need to help an employee, it's important that you remind yourself that you can't "move" the employee to where they experience being in control of their life. You can help them, but they have to do the work for themselves. This involves developing strategies to get back to the experience of being in control.

The locus of control model also provides an understanding of why sick leave isn't always appropriate when things start to become difficult. Imagine you have an employee showing symptoms of stress. They experience not being in control. Then they get sick. Does sick leave bring them closer to developing strategies for how to deal with what is difficult for them? No, it doesn't. Here, sick leave equates to removing a burden (one of the arrows pointing to the employee on the right side of the figure). It may well feel like an immediate relief, but it rarely helps them regain the fundamental experience of being in control of their own life.

HOW TO HELP AN EMPLOYEE REGAIN CONTROL
Talk about solutions and ask:

- Do you have any suggestions of your own for what could help?
- Would you like to hear my suggestion for what you could do?
- So what is the concrete plan from here on?

If the experience of pressure is about work, then something as simple as setting up an automatic answer to emails for a few days can be a solution that helps the employee who is behind in their work. But keep in mind that while the extra time bought by setting up an automated answer can be helpful, it is the *experience* of being able to do something that makes everything come together more positively that makes the big difference, not the action itself. Perhaps you also discover that the employee needs to be able to put "go home at 3" into their diary every Wednesday, so they can be sure of driving their daughter to tennis. Or you might clearly agree that for a specific period of time, with a clear end-date, the employee works overtime to get through all their assignments.

Practical solutions can be all kinds of things, and when it comes down to it they don't always require a lot. But if, as managers, we aren't aware of providing the right help and support in time, the employee's symptoms of stress can worsen and they may find themselves being unfairly treated. That leads us to the next key concept in Step 3: fairness.

Fairness takes up a lot of time

What does something being fair or unfair really mean? If something is fair, most people will experience it as being reasonable. But fairness is an individual experience. For example, most people would agree that it's reasonable for criminals to be punished. But for those convicted, going to jail might feel unreasonable or unfair.

When we talk about fairness in connection with the workplace, it often has something to do with the relationship between employee and manager. Sentiments such as "It's so unfair that my manager always praises my colleague for her work while she hardly notices mine" and "It's not fair that it's always me who gets the late shift on Fridays" are very common. Again here, fairness is connected to individual interpretation.

An employee's experience of fairness can also be put to the test if they experience an entire system as being unfair. Perhaps they don't think the new changes at work are reasonable. No matter who they perceive as their adversary – whether it be you as a manager, the workplace, the system or something else – the experience of unfairness can lead to symptoms of stress (see the lists in Step 1).

Many managers aren't aware that employees' symptoms of stress can essentially be about feeling unfairly treated. When an employee says they can't manage something, it might not have anything to do with the new task at hand. They might believe that something is unfair at work, but the manager can't see what it is – on the contrary, they might even think that a given situation is very fair.

Today, we know that if an employee experiences their work as unclear or unfair it can have major consequences. We know too that there's a significantly greater correlation between the psychological working environment and stress-related disorders than we believed previously. It's not always the piles of paper on our desks that make us sick. This became apparent in a 2007-2009 study from Aarhus in which a total of 4,500 public sector employees participated. Here, stress-related disorders such as depression and anxiety (ref. 17, 18) were evident among subjects and led to a higher rate of absence due to sickness when the subjects experienced being unfairly treated by their managers. The same thing happened if their work and/or work processes suddenly became unclear. The subjects then became sick with stress. While those who experienced their workplaces as being fair and transparent when it came to organising work became *less* ill with stress-related diseases.

Now you are going to meet an employee who illustrates what the study concluded.

Unfairness broke her

Mary's story

59-year-old Mary has been working as a cleaning assistant in a municipality for years. She's hardly ever missed a day's work due to illness, despite being a single mother of two boys. But suddenly Mary begins sleeping badly at night. She got a new boss and a new, younger colleague. It's her new manager's first managerial position and he's so green behind the ears that Mary has difficultly communicating with him. It's the same story with the new colleague. But the colleague and the boss communicate with each other easily, which makes Mary feel left out. Previously, Mary's work was assessed every six months, but now it's happening once a month or more often. The new boss walks around, smartphone lit up, to check on the places Mary has cleaned. She gradually becomes more and more uncertain about whether or not she's doing her job well enough. It makes her feel insecure. She feels monitored and as if she isn't trusted. At the same time, she has noticed that her colleague isn't being checked as much, and this surprises Mary, because the new colleague isn't doing her job properly, and she doesn't get as much done as Mary either. Mary experiences the work processes as being unclear and unfair.

After a while, Mary's boss calls her in for a chat. He would like to talk to her about how she could work more effectively. Mary doesn't know what to say. She starts crying and can't stop. Her boss suggests that Mary takes a few days off. Mary does as he says. But once the days have passed, Mary isn't any better. Quite the opposite. She ends up going on long-term sick leave. The doctor says Mary is depressed, and that it was brought on by stress.

New boss, new routines

Most people change managers and colleagues many times during their working lives. And today many people experience their work being evaluated much more than before. We have to document almost everything now in practically every industry. There is nothing wrong with documentation in itself and documentation doesn't necessarily have to lead to stress-related sick leave either. It's a question of *how* it's done.

Many employees within the healthcare sector are currently experiencing that the increased focus on evaluations is putting them under pressure as it takes time away from their core work. Maybe they perceive the assessments as meaningless. Perhaps they even experience the system as unfair. It is precisely when these experiences arise that we must be aware of what they do to our employees. Mary and all the other employees bear a responsibility to inform their managers when an experience of unfairness occurs and when something isn't as it should be. But it's difficult if that kind of culture hasn't been created and you, as the manager, aren't attentive and responsive to what may be going on behind the immediate reactions.

It may well be that Mary ends up being depressed, but in the beginning her experience of unfairness is expressed as difficulty concentrating, trouble sleeping and worrying . . . And she experiences being isolated from the community that her new colleague shares with the new boss. Depression develops because the symptoms are allowed to develop over time.

Fairness is a two-way street

You can also experience unfairness as a manager. Many managers find that sometimes it can be difficult to stay on the riverbank as we talked about in Step 2, if an employee reacts in a way that is unfair or unreasonable in the manager's eyes. For example, perhaps you have seen and acknowledged changes in an employee's behaviour. You have asked all the right questions at the right time. You know what it's all about – the employee is experiencing a form of unfairness at work and is having difficulty letting it go. Even if you don't agree about the situation being unfair, you have suggested several concrete solutions and really gone the extra mile. But the employee just isn't satisfied and their negative attitude continues. You know the employee isn't doing it on purpose and you try to hold on to the knowledge that we humans quite often get annoyed when we experience being under pressure. It's not about your employee, but rather about the situation. No matter what you do, you and the employee can't reach a common understanding on how to proceed and find a solution. Fuses are short. Colleagues are complaining. It's heading in only one direction, and you can almost see the sick leave on the horizon. What do you do?

Let's see what a manager in this situation did.

Enough is enough!

Mark is one of the top managers of his organisation. One Friday afternoon he sticks his head into his employee Edward's office and wishes him a nice weekend. Edward lifts his head up from his desk and looks Mark straight in the eye, but doesn't say anything. Instead, he turns his gaze to the screen in front of him.

"Have a nice weekend," repeats Mark, still without getting a reply.

Mark marches directly into his shared managers' office and tells them how tired he is of Edward. For two weeks now he's been trying to draw up a project plan that matches Edward's wishes and expectations, but no matter what he does, Edward is dissatisfied. And now he won't even return a greeting.

"I understand that you're getting annoyed," reassures his managerial colleague. "I would be, too. But I wonder why Edward is reacting like this? He doesn't usually do that. Can you find out what it's all about?"

After chewing on that for a moment, Mark goes back to Edward's office.

"How are things going?"

Edward looks up, surprised.

"What do you mean?"

"Is everything all right with you?" Mark asks.

Edward sighs angrily and returns to the papers he was working on.

"I just want to have some peace and quiet to work! It's not easy trying to finish stuff when you're always being interrupted."

"I can understand that. But it seems as if something is going on, and I'd like to help you if that's the case. You just have to tell me what's wrong. Has one of your projects run into difficulty? You and I made a new plan last week, but if that's not working, you should tell me so we can find out how I can help you."

Mark tries to remain calm and collected. Inside, he's seething, but he knows reacting like that won't do any good. They have to find out what this is all about. What has caused the cogs to run so awry that they can hardly talk to each other? And how can they fix it again?

Edward is obviously annoyed and hesitant to talk to Mark, who is very tempted to leave again. Mark thinks about what will happen if they don't have a proper talk before the weekend. Will Edward end up on sick leave? Or will he want to look for a new job?

"Look, I can hear you're frustrated about something. I don't think I fully understand what it is, and I don't know if it's me you're angry with, but we have to talk about it," says Mark.

Edward's attitude seems to change. "I don't really know . . ." he says. "I just feel like I'm doing everything on my own, and it's like you're not taking me seriously when I tell you how difficult it all is. You're not the one the customer calls when we don't deliver what was agreed." He pauses briefly before continuing. "I know that you don't understand everything I do and that's okay . . . I just need you to understand that it's actually pretty hard to get it all done sometimes and that I'm doing my best."

Mark notices a clear breakthrough in the conversation. He acknowledges Edward's openness and says it's definitely something he will be aware of in the future. Mark does actually understand how Edward feels. It's undoubtedly easier for him to understand and praise those employees whose jobs and workloads are similar to his. Edward and Mark then talk about what

Edward needs, and they agree that he should use auto-reply on his email for a few days, so he can catch up on a few things. They also agree to meet the following Tuesday to talk about how they are going to work together and their expectations of each other, and to outline the plan for the project.

During the conversation, Edward reveals that he is feeling pressure from several sides. His girlfriend moved out two weeks ago. Edward himself admits that his change in behaviour probably has something to do with that.

An hour later, and both feeling better, they head home for the weekend.

When Mark gets into his car, he is tired. But he's also a little proud of himself. It would have been easy for him to give in to the anger he felt when Edward hadn't initially wanted to talk to him and was obviously angry. Mark thought it was difficult to stay on the riverbank when he was exposed to so much unwarranted negativity from Edward. But now he knows that with professional curiosity, it's possible to get the cogs to align again. He didn't let himself be bested by his feelings, but insisted on understanding the situation.

Don't add fuel to the unfairness fire

Sometimes, when, as managers, we avoid having conversations with our employees about their experience of unfairness, it is because we can't or won't change the situation. We may be looking at the group as a whole and believe that there are no better solutions. Why talk to an employee if we can't change anything anyway?

In the story of Mark and Edward, Mark doesn't step in and change anything in Edward's work. Mark still doesn't really understand what Edward does, and even though Edward feels pressured, Mark doesn't take any assignments from him. But Mark does take Edward seriously. He listens to him and his perspective and promises to be aware of the unfairness he experiences when he witnesses his colleagues getting more praise than him.

When a feeling of unfairness is allowed to fester, without being addressed or taken seriously, it can cause symptoms of stress. Here, the employee is pushed into the experience of control lying outside their influence, and feeling that they can't do anything about it. Even if you don't or can't agree with your employee, you can easily talk to them about the fact that they are experiencing something as difficult and unfair and that they would like things to be otherwise. As a manager, you can be curious, take such concerns seriously and acknowledge that this is how your employee is feeling. And, of course, you can investigate whether you can help the employee gain a sense of control, despite a decision being made that they don't agree with. The most important thing is that you don't *avoid* the conversation on unfairness due to it being uncomfortable. If that happens, you will have added fuel to the unfairness fire.

Stress from private life affects us in the workplace

Most managers know that an employee's burden is sometimes wholly or partly due to personal matters. We saw this in the example of Edward. But should you, as a manager, concern yourself with stress when it is due to factors in the employee's private life?

In a word: yes. As we mentioned earlier, it's always better to ask than not to. We are humans, not machines. It's crucial that, as workplaces and managers, we give space to employees dealing with emotions and reacting if something in their life is difficult. Perhaps something has gone wrong at home. Perhaps it's at work. Most people experience both. That's why the sharp divide between work and home doesn't work in practice. We spend hours and hours at work. So if we're under pressure, the workplace has to be part of the solution – regardless of the reasons. The next story is an example of this.

The workplace is part of the solution

Martin's story

When Martin, who is a star worker at one of the country's largest organisations in the financial sector, finds out that his six-year-old son has autism, he is hugely affected and experiences it as a great burden. His son receiving such a diagnosis puts him under pressure and affects his work. He can no longer concentrate, he forgets appointments and both his appetite and his good mood go down the drain. He no longer shares anecdotes with his colleagues at lunch, but just sits quietly at the table while the others eat. He sleeps badly at night and that is affecting his ability to work.

Fortunately, Martin's manager is aware of this, so she takes Martin aside after just a week of symptoms and reactions.

"What's happened?" asks the manager as they sit in her office with the door closed.

Martin hesitates and looks down at his hands. Then he tells her about his son's diagnosis.

"Autism? What does that mean?" she asks. Deliberately, she says neither that she understands Martin nor that she pities him. She speaks in the same tone of voice as she usually does – curious, sincere and professional.

Martin explains what autism is and where on the scale his son probably lies. They don't yet know for sure; his son has to go through more tests.

"What's putting the most pressure on you right now?" the manager asks.

"Uncertainty," replies Martin, and then they talk a little about the upheaval it's going to cause for his family, and about his son's probable needs for extra support and more structure.

"Is there something we can do so that things are easier for you?" the manager asks.

Martin tells her about all the meetings with the educational, and the social and health services that he and his wife are being called to at the moment. Sometimes several times a week. He feels like he has lost all control over his life and his diary. When sitting in meetings with case workers and autism experts, he thinks about work: how can he cope? And will things ever be normal again? And when he's at work, he thinks about his son: what's going to happen to his son? And to them as a family? At the same time, Martin is concerned about how it will affect his career and what others will think of him if he doesn't perform as he usually does.

The manager proposes a temporary flexible arrangement so that Martin can prioritise the meetings about his son in good conscience. Just until things calm down at home. Martin says that he and his wife have already discussed whether it is necessary for both of them to attend all the meetings. They have talked about making a long-term plan where Martin and his wife will take turns to deal with everything related to their son in alternate weeks. His manager thinks this sounds like a good plan. But it doesn't solve the specific work pressure that will probably arise now, while Martin prioritises getting things at home under control.

"Are there any assignments or projects you can postpone? Or possibly hand over to one of your colleagues?" asks the manager.

Martin thinks for a while. Handing over some of the projects to someone else won't help, but two out of the five projects could be postponed.

His manager nods. That's a deal. They also agree for Martin

to update the manager every Monday, so she can follow developments, and she promises to be open about her expectations of him so that he doesn't have to worry about whether or not she is satisfied with his work.

In the time that follows, it remains clear that there is something weighing on Martin. He is upset for his son and his family. Temporary less strict conditions at work don't remove the diagnosis. But his flexible work hours and manager's support in postponing two projects helps Martin get through a difficult time without worsening his symptoms of stress.

As a manager, you can never remove challenges from the employee's private life – and nor is that your job. But you can help the employee find a practical solution that prevents them from taking sick leave to cope with what is putting pressure on them. As a rule, the workplace is part of the solution. And therefore, stress in an employee's private life concerns the workplace.

Now you're going to see a workplace where the manager doesn't intervene in the same professional manner. Harriet's story illustrates how stress in an employee's private life concerns the workplace, but in contrast to Martin's manager, Harriet's manager decides at first to wait and see what happens. When she sees that this isn't the way forward, she intervenes, but she does so in a way that ends up making the situation worse.

Misplaced consideration

Harriet was once everyone's favourite. In the morning, all the children in the kindergarten threw their arms around her. The parents loved dropping off their little ones to her. But the manager has noticed that the parents are now seeking other arms for their children. She has also spotted the cool silence between Harriet and her colleagues at their staff meetings. Even when they're just drinking coffee. From colleagues, the manager hears about Harriet being cranky, critical and difficult to get along with. The manager thinks it's a difficult situation, because Harriet has been part of the day-care centre for more than eight years, so how is she supposed to handle it? The manager doesn't want to offend anyone.

Harriet hardly ever took a sick day before. But now she's had 24 days off in six months. That's more than an entire month. When that becomes clear to the manager, she decides to invite Harriet to have a chat. In the manager's office, Harriet suddenly breaks down.

"It's just so hard at home. With my husband, I mean. The doctors say it looks bad. I don't know what to do. I don't even know myself anymore. And I think my colleagues are out to get me. I just need to do things my way until I get a little more energy."

The manager takes Harriet's hand, squeezes it and says: "I can understand that. I'm here and I'm listening. And I'll make sure that the others take this into account until you're on your feet again."

Harriet's manager has good intentions. But the consideration she shows Harriet throughout the period actually helps reinforce the problem. Harriet hasn't been helped by her manager. The manager has shown clear avoidance behaviour. Harriet's levels of absence due to illness have been high for six months, and despite her manager talking to Harriet about her absences a few times and finding out that Harriet has had both influenza and pneumonia, she's never directly said to Harriet that she is experiencing changes in Harriet's behaviour. The manager thought that would have to wait until the period of sick leave was over. And now the obvious problem and Harriet's husband's illness have become even worse, so the manager doesn't feel she can talk about the changes. In other words, the manager has fewer options to influence the situation because she didn't intervene in time.

It can be difficult to be a manager when an employee is falling apart. Most people intuitively want to comfort the person sitting on the other side of the desk. It is here that the manager needs to be aware of remaining on the riverbank. The manager shouldn't be Harriet's understanding friend. And neither should she transform herself into a patiently listening therapist. The manager can't and shouldn't do anything about Harriet's husband's situation. What she should do is focus on helping Harriet find a practical solution to relieve the work pressure that has arisen over the situation with her husband's illness.

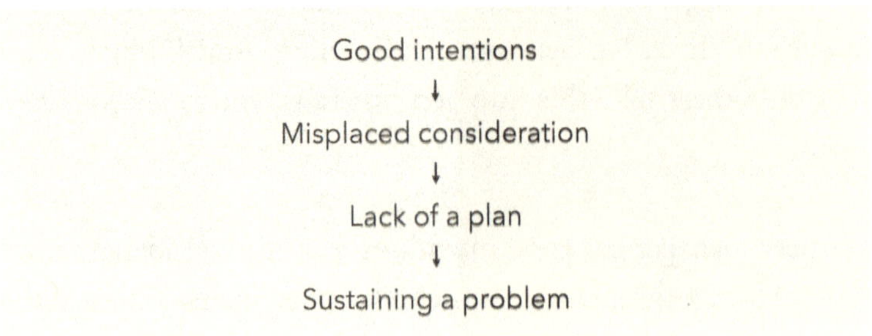

Set demands

Harriet needs a manager who will intervene and take the situation seriously. A manager who will acknowledge that Harriet is having a very hard time at home and who can accommodate Harriet's difficult emotions right now. She isn't a robot that can be turned on and off, but rather a person who brings her private life to work. And, of course, Harriet is finding it difficult with her husband being sick. Harriet needs a manager who is clear in her expectations of Harriet, and who says: "We need you here. The children need you. Your colleagues need you. This is a workplace, and we talk to each other properly here – even when life is tough. We need to find a solution where things work for you – and your colleagues."

MAKE A PLAN

A good manager is clear about their expectations and helps to make a plan:

"I understand that your current situation is difficult. But I expect you to talk nicely to your colleagues, no matter what is going on in your private life."

"I expect you to follow the agreement we've made. If something happens that changes the situation, I expect you to tell me so we can adapt the plan."

"I would like us to work on your levels of sick leave. They're very high. What would it take for us to reduce that?"

After the conversation with Harriet, some time passes before the manager calls a staff meeting. Here, she says to all the employees: "We've all noticed that the tone has changed somewhat here at work. Harriet is having a hard time. Her husband is very ill, and of course it's affecting Harriet. I want to encourage everyone to bear with her so she's able to cope with the difficult situation at home."

The manager informs the department about what is at stake, which is positive despite it happening late in the process.

It is, however, not positive that the manager gives the green light to the behaviour Harriet has been exhibiting for more than six months, and that she asks the employees to be understanding about this behaviour.

In the time that follows, Harriet doesn't get any better. Her behaviour and tone remain problematic, and her level of absence is unchanged. It's beginning to affect the other employees. Some are taking sick days too. Others ask to change rooms so they can avoid working directly with Harriet. More and more parents are giving the impression that they would like their child in a room other than Harriet's too, if possible. The manager's desk turns into a jigsaw puzzle of children, staff and hours that all need to fit together. She doesn't focus on the development and strategy of the day-care centre at all. Finally, the situation in the department is so tense that Harriet goes on full-time sick leave due to stress. After four months she is fired.

Harriet's story clearly illustrates how early symptoms of stress can develop into inappropriate patterns, problematic behaviour and sick leave. And how difficult it can be if you don't intervene in time. Things didn't have to go so wrong with Harriet. Harriet has always been a popular employee, but now she is left with a husband who is seriously ill, a group of colleagues who don't like her and she has lost her job. The manager thought she was helping Harriet, but it's precisely because she felt sorry for Harriet that she failed in her duty as a manager. She was understanding and tolerant, but forgot to be aware, professionally curious and clear in her expectations. She didn't help Harriet make a plan for how she could be a good employee when she was at work. In other words, she didn't help Harriet regain control, but left her with the experience of powerlessness and frustration – in her work too. Harriet's manager would probably argue that making demands when Harriet is having such a difficult time at home doesn't show empathy. Unfortunately, the story shows how, as managers, if we fail to make demands, it can quickly have the opposite effect.

Trouble in paradise

David's story

David often works late into the night. He's often the last one to leave the office, and although it sometimes gets quite late, he is fine with that, because he likes to get things completely finished and he is always thorough. David has a girlfriend whom he is very fond of, but she has a problem with how he is prioritising his work over her. She starts complaining and it rubs off on David. David's manager soon notices a shift in David. David makes many more mistakes than he normally would. He looks tired. And his mood has also changed. The David who always had plenty of time for his colleagues is suddenly more concerned with what is on his desk.

The manager wonders about this and calls David in to talk. He shares his observations and asks if there's anything he should be aware of as David's manager. David doesn't really know what to say. Should he really involve his manager in the fact that his girlfriend is tired of his job? He chooses to start with something completely different and points out that the photocopier often plays up. And that one of their suppliers often makes mistakes. Finally, he admits that he thinks it's difficult to balance doing everything and that he feels inadequate when, on the one hand, there are exciting assignments on his desk that he would like to get under control, but at the same time knows that his girlfriend will be disappointed and angry if he comes home late yet again.

"Yes, I can see that," says his manager. "It's a dilemma. So, what do you think is needed to solve the situation? Is there anything I can do to help?"

David shakes his head. He doesn't know. His work means a lot to him – but so does his girlfriend.

He says that his girlfriend dreams of at least one evening a week when they make dinner and eat together – without telephones and work emails alongside them. The manager ponders this. Is David really always available on email? He's never asked that his staff reply to emails or calls in the evening. It must be David placing these demands on himself, creating an issue because of how he is interpreting the situation. If the manager doesn't succeed in leading David in a better direction, then over time David will go under. Either his girlfriend will leave him, or he will get overwhelmed by the work habits he has created for himself. But his manager can't and won't interfere in David's relationship with his girlfriend. That isn't his job and he won't become David's couple's therapist either. But he can help David with his experience of work pressure and the lack of boundaries in relation to his work.

David's manager suggests that David begins to structure his work more strictly so that he doesn't have to work every night. For example, he can mark in his diary that three days a week he finishes work at 4 pm, while he can allow himself to work as long as he wants the other days.

David thinks this sounds like a slightly silly solution. And also a little obvious. Is he really unable to manage his own time? He's ashamed, but agrees to give it a try.

A few weeks later, David tells his manager that his suggestion has had a major effect. He is experiencing that he has gained more of an overview of his everyday life. As an aside, he says that his girlfriend has already asked what happened to him, because she can feel a difference. He is smiling. His manager can also see that the work-related errors that had crept into David's projects have disappeared. He is himself again – without having taken a single sick day.

David's story shows how concrete and practical stress prevention management can be. Often, it's about having a curious approach and using your common sense. In principle, it's easy to help create structure and set a framework like David's manager does. It simply requires that, as a manager, you view stress in a different way than the traditional one you may be used to. As we mentioned earlier, stress isn't just about too much work – it's very much about thoughts and feelings; for example, the experience of control and unfairness described in this section.

So when, as a manager, you need to prevent stress, it's a good idea to choose to move away from your avoidance behaviour. First, you need to be professionally curious and interested in the employee's experience. Once you understand that, you can help find a practical solution that can assist your employee to return to an experience of being in control of their situation.

FIND THE SOLUTION - IN SHORT

- Be particularly aware of the experience of unfairness.
- Be clear about your expectations and don't be afraid to set demands.
- Remember: small practical changes at work can have a huge effect.
- Work with your employee to find a concrete solution – and try it out.
- Insist that you make a plan together that helps the employee achieve an experience of control.

One of the reasons a manager isn't often more insistent with an employee who isn't thriving is the fear of pushing the employee too much, so they end up worse. Many managers have huge concerns about the serious consequences a conversation with the employee could have.

There's no guarantee that what you are trying will succeed. But the consequences of being inactive and not making a plan can be far more serious than the consequences of being active and direct. It's about being active in an appropriate way based on a real desire to help the employee to gain control. You have to be sure of your intention with the conversation. Then you can more easily deal with your fear of getting too close.

An employee on sick leave has the right to refuse that you, as a manager, say anything to their colleagues, and, in principle, you can't change that. But try to urge the employee on sick leave to accept that you are sharing relevant information about the situation with their colleagues. This will give colleagues a greater understanding of the situation, and they will find it easier to support the plan you have made with the employee. Perhaps the employee needs the openness around their situation to be limited, for example, by only telling the union representative, the working environment representative and some select colleagues. It would be nice if you and your employee agree on what is to be said and how – for example, in an email to colleagues. It's best if you tell them of the benefits of sharing relevant information with their colleagues *before* they go on sick leave, and that you urge them to do this.

My employee has been working here for a year and has been feeling under pressure since they started. They aren't satisfied. I can't change any more conditions for them. How do we move forward?

Management and leadership can be a delicate balance in some situations. How long do we need to develop and compensate – and when should we recognise that the employment conditions aren't working for either the employee or the employer? As a rule of thumb, you shouldn't make a drastic decision, for example, to dismiss an employee, who is sick and not receiving treatment. If the employee hasn't been receiving the necessary health care during the process, the prerequisite for assessing whether or not they are fit for their position isn't present.

It may be necessary to point out to an employee that you and the workplace are dependent on the employee's functional level increasing. The clearer you are about your expectations and demands for the position, and the more you regularly write down the things you have worked on to help the employee succeed, the clearer it will be when you have to make a choice. Remain standing on the riverbank, and talk openly with your employee about what they can do themselves and what the workplace can do. And set a follow-up deadline. If your employee continues to be dissatisfied and discontent after a number of relevant initiatives, and you have no more to offer, it will be important to talk about whether the employee should continue – for both the workplace and the employee's own sake. If there is absolutely no development, it will be necessary for you to be aware that you manage the individual employee's interests on the one hand, and the interests of the workplace and colleagues on the other.

My employee is showing symptoms of stress and they say it's my fault and that of the workplace that they aren't doing well. I think this is wrong and unfair.

The perception of unfairness can take up a lot of space and time, both for the employee and the manager, and it's associated with emotions that, to a great extent, can cause us to jump into the metaphorical river. It's in those situations that you really need to hold onto your professional curiosity. Why is the employee feeling like this? What concrete examples is the employee providing? How do you experience the employee's interpretation of the situation? Try to set aside your own feelings and concentrate on the employee's experience. You can hold onto your own experience of the situation while acknowledging the employee's.

When that is done, you will be better able to make a plan. Be honest about the available options, but also about the demands and expectations of the position. Investigate whether there are places where you can improve the conditions for the employee, but be clear about the things that can't be changed. If, for example, the employee is a child-care worker and thinks it's unreasonable for them to take the late shift, it's important that you are honest about the need for you to share the task so that they can continue in their job.

It can't always be denied that, as a manager, you may have had an unfortunate influence on an employee. The behaviour of some managers can cause their employees stress. Fortunately, we rarely experience managers who deliberately bring about discomfort in their employees. There is a risk that your behaviour will be perceived as stress-inducing by an employee, no matter how much effort you make. The less time that passes before you both talk about it, the less risk of affirming the employee's experience that you are at the root of their stress.

FOLLOW-UP

Pay attention to whether or not the solution
you have reached with the employee is helping.
And whether it's sustainable.

There is almost always a need for a follow up
- initially, a close follow up and then at longer
intervals. This helps keep the focus on what you
both agreed and helps avoid a return to stress.

Keep regular and informal contact with the
employee. Telephone often, meet often.
But you also need to prioritise the more
formal wellbeing interview.

You will get to know your employee
better, which in turn will lead to a better
working partnership in the long run.

MAINTAIN CONTACT

It's one thing to pick up on behavioural changes, step in and make a good plan. It's something else entirely to maintain that plan and ensure that development is moving in the right direction. Everyday life quickly takes over, and there's a major risk that both you and your employee will return to old habits. If we continue to do the same thing, we get the same result. There is a great risk that our avoidance behaviour will once again intervene – it's always biding its time because it's such a natural part of human behaviour – which can lead to us doubting whether a plan is sustainable in the long run. And that's a shame, because it's a waste of wonderful energy. If changes are to become new habits, they need to be followed up. Following up is crucial for whether or not the specific solution or solutions initiated by you and your employee actually achieve the desired effect.

How good are you at following up on the plan that you made with your employee for preventing or limiting stress? Many managers believe it's important to prioritise following up – especially if it concerns an employee who has been, or is on the verge of going on, sick leave. But when we examine *how* individual managers and workplaces follow up on those employees showing early signs of stress, the results vary widely. Many admit that they don't get to follow up and so their agreements go out of the window – with the risk that the employee's stress will flare up again.

Some managers don't even consider the need to follow up. They sit back, content that a plan has now been made, and then they hope for the best after only one conversation. Other managers send an email to the employee now and again, often in relation to a specific work-related matter. You may think that repeatedly asking an employee directly about how things are going is showing too much curiosity, and so you sneak it into another "conversation" – in writing. The problem is that the effect of an email isn't the same as the effect of a phone call or a face-to-face conversation. When humans communicate in writing, it's a different experience than when we *talk* to each other.

Some managers are good at maintaining contact and asking the employee how things are going, but the conversations are neither structured nor planned systematically. They often happen randomly, for example, when the employee and manager bump into each other in the corridor or in the canteen, and the manager takes the opportunity to ask: "How are you?" The situation doesn't leave proper time to listen or answer, just as there is no time for follow-up questions either. So, the content of this kind of conversation develops unintentionally based on what the situation allows, and you don't get to talk about what you and the employee can do together to maintain the changes and what you can do to create an even better situation: is the work the problem? Should their work hours be reconsidered? Do they have too much or not enough responsibility? Or is it something else entirely that's not working or could work better? And lastly, there are also managers who confuse following up as needed with the annual employee appraisal interview. But in the context of stress-prevention, focus on an individual employee can't be reduced to an annual event. It's vital that the conversations happen continuously.

All this demonstrates that there is a lack of solid knowledge about following up. A method for following up systematically and consistently is needed. Here in the fourth and final part of the book, we describe two ways to follow up:

- Informal, frequent contact between employee and manager
- Formal wellbeing interviews

Each of the two follow-up methods has its own purpose. So it's important that you use the right method in the right situation. Common to both methods is that the manager is, firstly, aware of what they are doing and, secondly, doing it in a structured way – rather than as random meetings.

TWO WAYS TO FOLLOW UP
- Informal, frequent contact
- Formal wellbeing interviews

Informal, frequent contact between the employee and manager could, for example, be a phone call a few times a week. This method is useful if an employee is isolating themselves or if you have a feeling that the employee needs more of a helping hand for a while. It demands extra contact and attention. The phone call could take a while or be quite brief. It's the contact between the employee and manager that is the purpose of the call. Therefore, how long you talk for is unimportant and nor does the conversation need an actual agenda. The most important thing is that you have contact with the employee; that you listen to them and talk to them. That you show you are aware and are following them up more closely than usual. Quick, brief physical meetings, where you hear about the employee and their day, can also be useful here.

A **formal wellbeing interview** between the employee and manager could take place once every two weeks or once a month. You set aside about half an hour for the conversation between you and your employee. You meet one-to-one – for example, in your office – to emphasise the high priority of the conversation and talk about how things have been going since your last meeting. The purpose of the meeting is to take stock of the employee's workload, work hours and responsibilities. At the meeting, the time of the next meeting is also agreed. The structured format provides a sense of security and peace of mind for both you and the employee.

Facts rather than feelings

There is a risk that the follow-up conversation will start with you, as a manager, asking how things are going, after which the employee will respond with a "fine". What does that mean? It can be difficult for both of you to get something useful out of the follow-up conversation if it's unstructured and vague.

One way to structure follow-up conversations is to use what we call the FACT model. This model enables you to create a recognisable structure for both of you, so you know and can prepare for what you are going to talk about when you meet. The model ensures that you talk about what is important, and that you get to talk about how things have been going since you last spoke. When you use the model, you and the employee avoid "thinking" or "sensing" something that could swing the conversation depending on whether it's a good or bad day. The follow-up meeting will focus on facts rather than feelings.

The FACT model gives an overview of:
- Work hours
- Work duties
- Responsibility and expectations
- The next meeting

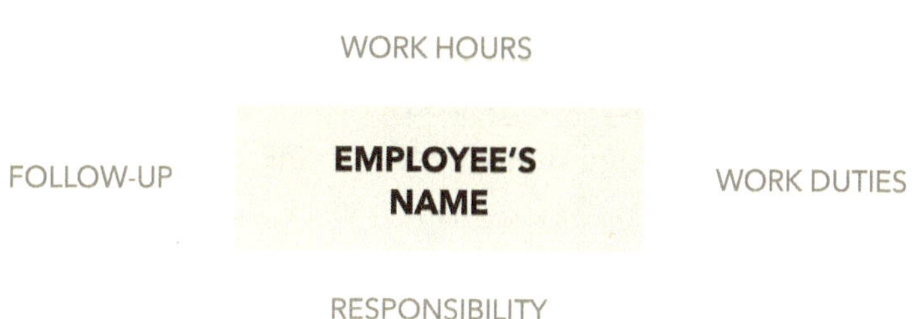

- **Name**

    Begin by writing the employee's name in the centre of a diagram. The name framed clearly in the middle signifies that boundaries are being set around the employee. This is simple, but many people experience it as a useful tool precisely because setting boundaries can be difficult for the individual employee.

- **Work hours**

    Talk to the employee about their work hours so you are both clear on when the employee will come to work in the period before you meet again. As they are regaining the experience of control and stability, it's vital that the employee not be left to assess for themselves how long they can or should be at work on a daily basis. This entails a risk that the subject will play on the employee's conscience, and so affect how long they will stay at work. It rarely results in the desired stability, but rather in a pattern of fluctuating work days, where the employee works too long for a few days and then needs to recuperate for a few days afterwards. Write the employee's concrete working hours for the coming period in the top box of the diagram. How many hours is the employee going to work? And what are those hours exactly?

- **Work duties**

    Make it clear which work duties the employee is to prioritise so that they aren't solely responsible for judging what is most important and what can wait. For example, ask the employee to make a list of all their work duties and then use that list to evaluate and prioritise together what is important and realistic for the employee to do within the stated working hours. Note the employee's specific work duties for the coming period in the box on the right.

- **Responsibility and expectations**
  Talk about what responsibility the employee is expected to take on for the chosen work duties. For example, where is the employee to go if something unexpected happens that creates problems? Or if a colleague doesn't deliver what is needed to move forward or if the schedule changes? Note who is responsible for what, so it's clear to the employee when they can ask for help and who they should go to.

- **Follow-up**
  Agree on when you are going to meet again and note it on the left side of the diagram. Add the meeting to your diary, too. An employee will often be more comfortable approaching work duties and hours when they know exactly when you are going to talk again and can adjust the plan if it becomes too challenging.

This model gets what can be difficult to talk about and relate to out of your head and down onto paper. When you work with appointments and follow-up based on a visual figure, the process becomes manageable. You get an overview and can prioritise, and you avoid getting bogged down in emotions. The model ensures that you and your employee talk about the same thing in the same way every time you meet. This makes it easier for you to remain on the metaphorical riverbank. There are fewer misunderstandings and greater openness.

In the following case story, you are going to meet a business where the manager doesn't initially use follow-up as a conscious management method. But then everything goes wrong. The employee breaks down. So the manager begins to use follow-up more consistently and systematically, which changes the course of the situation.

Good start, but no follow through

Marie's story

"This just has to stop now. I won't be part of this any more if they continue with all their unreasonable demands!"

With tears in her eyes, Marie stormed out of her boss, Jim's, office. She was furious with a customer who kept making new demands and who repeatedly questioned the solutions they had previously agreed on. It had been like that for almost a year. Marie worked as an IT specialist and was good at her job. Both she and Jim knew it. But with this customer, it was as though no matter what she did it was never right – the customer continued to find errors and shortcomings, and had repeatedly denied agreeing to things that Marie had spent days and evenings – even nights – developing solutions based on. When she would then present the customer with the solution, they would say it wasn't at all what they'd had in mind and they would ask her to come up with something else.

Jim could clearly see that Marie had begun to change. She was smiling less, didn't go for her normal lunch breaks and seemed tired. When she'd stormed out of his office that day, he knew something was wrong. He'd never seen her lose her cool or be so angry. He went to find Marie, who was crying in her office.

"Look, don't worry about it. We'll find a solution. I think

I should come to the meetings with the customer in the short term, and we should work together on the project. I don't think they're behaving fairly either."

Marie continued to sob with her head in her hands.

"Are you okay, Marie?" Jim asked gently.

When Marie was able to speak again, she told Jim she had started to sleep badly, and that in the week leading up to a presentation to the customer, she'd hardly slept at all. She had lost her appetite and was apathetic. She had started thinking she was no good at her job, and had even gone so far as to seriously consider changing jobs completely. She began to cry again.

Jim and Marie agreed that Marie should take it easy and go home early for a while, so she could rest or go for a run before her children got home. They also agreed to collaborate on the difficult customer's project, like Jim proposed.

After just a week, Marie was feeling better. Jim and Marie ate lunch together, and Marie told him she had started to sleep better and had a bit more energy. They ate lunch together the following week too, and Marie said she was now back to her old self. Jim was happy. And satisfied with his efforts. He'd acted quickly, and that was apparently enough for Marie to experience that she was in control again.

Then weeks passed during which Marie and Jim hardly saw each other. Jim was tied up in meetings abroad and was essentially not in the office. He had difficulty getting to the meetings with the tricky customer as he had promised Marie, but he convinced both himself and Marie that she was perfectly able to handle the meetings on her own. Marie was a little hesitant, but agreed:

"Yes, I can do it. I shouldn't really be bringing someone to my meetings anyway. I should be able to do it myself."

"Where's Marie?" Jim asked when he came back after another trip abroad. He could see that Marie wasn't in her office.

"She's been off sick for a few days," replied a colleague. "She didn't look too good when she was here last time – might be the flu."

Jim felt that he didn't believe the flu explanation. He quickly rang Marie, but she didn't answer. He called several more times during the day, but she didn't pick up. Jim began to worry.

That evening he got an email from Marie. She wrote that she was sorry to have taken sick leave. She had thought she could handle it, but during the meeting with the challenging customer she had suddenly had difficulty breathing and had to cut the meeting short. The customer had become angry and she had heard him mutter the word "unprofessional" on his way out of the door. Marie apologised to Jim and wrote that she would understand if he chose to dismiss her as a consequence of this.

Jim was annoyed. With himself. And embarrassed. Inside, he knew perfectly well that Marie had been feeling under pressure. She had got a little less stressed, but hadn't recovered enough to deal with the difficult customer on her own. He had promised to support her, but he hadn't really done so. He had been so busy that he had crossed his fingers and hoped everything was going as it should. And now she was at home, obviously very unwell. He wrote back immediately, and they agreed to meet the next day.

It took a few weeks to convince Marie she should come back to work in the department. She'd lost both her confidence in herself and in Jim's support. But eventually she agreed to try. Marie and Jim now started every week by structurally following up together on her work hours, work duties and her areas of responsibility in projects. When they met, they talked concretely about who would be her sounding board when something became difficult while working with a customer, or if her responsibility became unclear. Their meetings were always held in Jim's office, and at the end of each meeting they agreed on when they were going to meet again.

After a month and a half, Marie was better again, but Jim insisted that they should keep up the follow-up meetings for another few months. Initially, they met every week, but gradually it became every other week. And finally just once a month.

Don't overestimate a stressed employee

You may be wondering whether it's really your place to sit and draw up such a simple model with one of your skilled employees. Maybe you just need to talk about the plan, and then your employee will get better. This was also what Jim first thought in Marie's story. But be careful not to overestimate an employee who is presenting with symptoms of stress. Whether or not your employee is professionally skilled, intelligent and a grown and responsible person has nothing to do with it. When we begin showing symptoms of stress, we don't think as well or as clearly as we usually do, and the risk of not making good, rational choices for ourselves increases. We've difficulty remembering and struggle more to get an overview of the situation. We become inclined to think "black and white". Like in the story when Marie starts thinking she's not good at anything at all.

When, as managers, we *don't* have the follow-up conversations, for example because we don't believe it to be necessary, or because we would like to signal to the employee that we trust they have things under control, we do neither the employee nor ourselves a favour. Actually, we risk throwing away all the good work we have done in relation to stress prevention.

By working with such a concrete and simple model, we can help the employee to create structure, remember agreements and get an overview of the situation. The employee can use the diagram later on their own. And by continuously following up, as a manager, you won't just be hoping that things are going well – you will be taking active responsibility for ensuring that this is actually the case.

FOLLOW-UP - IN SHORT

- Overcome your fear of getting too personal – be present and be visible.
- Make a plan for following-up. Make sure to keep in regular contact – agree, for example, to speak once a week for a while. And then at longer and longer intervals. Then schedule another meeting after a few months.
- Follow-up clearly: always agree on when you are going to meet again before ending a conversation.
- Talk about when things can be considered normal again, so, you don't remain overly watchful of an employee when it's no longer needed. That isn't in anyone's interest.

You can try to make contact – either in writing or by phone – but you can't demand that your employee talk to you before the formal meetings that the employee is called to. If the contact between you and your employee was already bad before they went on sick leave, or your employee is afraid of what you are going to say, it's difficult to make contact. But if you have made it clear to employees that it's company policy for the manager to ring an employee shortly after they go on sick leave and what you will talk about, then they will be prepared and will probably find the call less intimidating. Another option is to involve the union representative or the working environment representative and agree that one of them should contact the employee.

Remember that the goal isn't to push the employee back into work as quickly as possible, but to ensure that there is contact and that a plan is made so time doesn't just go by.

Entering into a dialogue with an employee whose therapist has discouraged it is a huge challenge. And it's not easy for you, as a manager, either, if you doubt a doctor's or psychologist's recommendation. A good piece of advice is to get the conversation going as early as possible. Make a plan for talking as soon as the employee takes sick leave. That way there's less risk of a therapist discouraging the dialogue. The therapist will also need to make an early and targeted effort to prevent the employee from getting worse.

It may be necessary to tell the employee how important it is to talk and to inform them of what can happen if you don't talk at all. Having guidelines implemented for regular conversations during the early phase of an employee's absence due to illness is of major advantage. That way the employee knows that this is normal in cases of stress-related sick leave and the contact won't surprise the employee, just as they will be able to better understand that you are doing it with good intentions.

If an employee takes sick leave for an indefinite period of time, you should talk to the employee about the undesirable situation and also try to achieve a constructive dialogue with their doctor about what would best serve the employee's interests, and whether a qualified estimate of the duration of sick leave can be given. Achieving such a dialogue can be a great challenge. Being given a statement of fitness for work is intended as a tool for getting started with the communication between you as the manager, your employee and the doctor.

My employee has symptoms of stress. We have made a few agreements, but they aren't sticking to them. How do I tackle this?

There is a balance between agreements, demands and mutual expectations that may need to be addressed. It might be important to emphasise that the agreements you make aren't only for the employee's own sake, but also for the sake of the workplace. If an employee has symptoms of stress, and you agree, for example, that they should finish at three o'clock every day and that isn't being respected, it's important to ask why the employee is choosing to do something else. You need to use your professional curiosity here. Your employee may be feeling that they should be achieving more than they can by 3 pm, and they may believe you think the same. However, your goal with the agreement is to help them become stable so they can regain the experience of control and get their time and work duties under control. The dialogue and clarification of expectations are crucial for the success of what you have agreed.

It's so busy at work that there's no time to do anything to prevent stress. Actually, top management isn't sympathetic to stress-related problems. So what are we supposed to do?
If there is persistent busyness at work that no one tackles and employees experience unfair working conditions, you have a particularly important, but also difficult, task as a manager. The top management of any workplace must participate in and take ownership of working with stress prevention management. Otherwise, there is a risk of it being all talk and no action and an immediate danger that as a manager, you will be caught between the stress developing in your employees and the demands for efficiency from above. And that experience could end up giving you stress in turn. In this book, we focus on the importance of the employee's experience of different situations, but we always have to take an interest in the objective burden and the consequences it can have. And satisfactory working conditions are, of course, a vital factor for both your own and your employees' wellbeing.

AFTERWORD

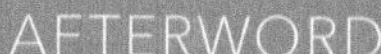

REMEMBER YOUR OWN MANAGERIAL BRAINSTORMING

Throughout the book, we have focused on how you can help your employees move away from stress. But where do you go for a sounding board and advice when you are in doubt and feel under pressure? Or when you don't know how to act towards an employee? Stress prevention management isn't just about the relationship and communication between you, as a manager, and your employee. It's also very much about you, your energy levels and your wellbeing. Who helps and guides you when you are facing challenges?

Many workplaces spend time and resources on creating a transparent chain of command for employees. But when it comes to the management team, what you do when you experience pressure or are feeling trapped in a difficult situation is often quite unclear. We recommend that you and the management team talk about who you go to. How does the chain of command work? Do you go up a level? Do you go to a managerial colleague? Or do you go to HR for support and brainstorming? It's difficult to avoid the informal competition between managers in most organisations. Therefore, many managers find that in reality openness doesn't apply to them in the same way as it applies to their employees. We encourage you to talk about what opportunities you have as managers for when challenges arise.

WHO HELPS YOU WHEN YOU ARE EXPERIENCING PRESSURE?
- Do you go to your own manager?
- Do you talk to a managerial colleague?
- Do you go up a few levels in the hierarchy?
- What does HR provide? How do you use HR?
- Do you have the opportunity to consult someone outside the organisation?

When should you be particularly aware of yourself?

From consulting with managers – and from our own experience as managers – we know, as we have previously mentioned, how difficult it can be to stay on the riverbank in relation to an employee. Remaining curious, open and professional isn't typically something a manager can just do – it requires training and awareness of themselves and their own reactions. Many of the managers we talk to recognise that they sometimes jump into the river with an employee. But with the help of colleagues, their own manager, consulting fellow managers or talking to HR, they are able to reach the bank again and be a good manager for that individual employee.

You need to pay particular attention when you find that an employee irritates you, angers you, frustrates you, upsets you or arouses your pity. Those emotions stand in the way of your professional curiosity and can lead to inappropriate emotional outbursts or misunderstandings. These emotions can reduce your power to act.

Throughout the book we've tried to illustrate, using stories, how managers have worked to achieve and maintain professional curiosity so their own personal opinions and feelings haven't got in the way. You *can't* avoid feeling something when you are facing an employee who, for example, is frustrated. In that situation, you can easily end up thinking it's your fault, despite you viewing the situation quite differently. But you can practise stepping back and examining your reactions and you can work on understanding what is happening.

It's not only important that you practise this in order to be a good manager for your employees and work actively with stress prevention management. It's also crucial to ensure that you personally experience job satisfaction, have a clear overview and maintain your energy levels.

READING LIST

1. Pedersen, P.S. *Udkast til et nyt copingbegreb: en kvalifikation af ledelsesmuligheder for at forebygge sygefravær ved psykiske problemer.* Frederiksberg: Copenhagen Business School [PhD thesis] 2016. (PhD Series, No. 05-2016). [A potential new coping mechanism: qualifying the opportunities of management to prevent absence due to mental health issues]
2. Danskernes Sundhed, Den Nationale Sundhedsprofil, 2017. [Report on the health of Danes by the Danish Health Service]
3. Stress: are we coping? https://www.mentalhealth.org.uk/publications/stress-are-we-coping A report on the prevalence of stress in the UK and its implications.
4. 2014 Study by the American Psychological Association https://www.apa.org/news/press/releases/stress/2014/stress-report.pdf
5. Lazarus, R.S.; Folkman, S. *Stress, appraisal, and coping.* New York: Springer, 1984.
6. *Mental health is your business, Guidance for developing a workplace policy.* Equality and Human Rights Commission at https://www.equalityhumanrights.com/sites/default/files/mental-health-is-your-business-wales.pdf
7. *Work-related Stress, Depression or Anxiety Statistics in Great Britain 2017.* Health and Safety Executive at http://www.hse.gov.uk/statistics/causdis/stress.pdf
8. *Mental Health and the Workplace.* POST – Parliamentary Office of Science and Technology Post note number 422, 2012, at http://researchbriefings.parliament.uk/ResearchBriefing/Summary/POST-PN-422

9. Videncenter for Arbejdsmiljø, 2018. Måder at forstå stress på http://www.arbejdsmiljoviden.dk/Emner/Psykosocialt-arbejdsmiljo/Stress/Viden-om-stress/Maader-at-forstaa-stress-paa [Report on ways to understand stress by the Danish Working Environment Authority]

10. Holmes, T.H. & R.H. Rahe. (1967). 'The Social Readjustment Rating Scale.' *Journal of Psychosomatic Research* 11 (2): 213-8. doi:10.1016/0022-3999(67)90010-4. PMID 6059863.

11. Social Kapital – Gylling Olesen, Kristian; Thoft, Eva; Hasle, Peter; Søndergaard Kristensen, Tage (2008). Virksomhedens Sociale Kapital – hvidbog, Arbejdsmiljørådet, Copenhagen, 2008. [White paper on Social Capital by the Danish Working Environment Advisory Council]

12. Ingre, Michael. *P-hacking in academic research: a critical review of the job strain model and of the association between night work and breast cancer in women.* PhD thesis, 2017, Stockholm University.

13. Judge, T.A., Piccolo, R.F. and R. Ilies. 'The forgotten ones? The validity of consideration and initiating structure in leadership research.' *Journal of Applied Psychology* 2004 Feb; 1989 (1): 36-51.

14. Holt Larsen, Henry, Poulfelt, Flemming and Rikke K. Nielsen. *Ny dansk ledelse. Når ledere taler om ledelse: VL-analyse* 2015. Copenhagen Business School Open Archive. [New Danish Leadership. When managers talk about leadership and management]

15. Rugulies, R., Aust, B. and I.E. Madsen. 'Effort-reward imbalance at work and risk of depressive diseases. A systematic review and meta-analysis of prospective cohort studies.' *Scandinavian Journal of Work, Environment and Health* 2017; 43 (4): 294-306.

16. Rotter, J.B. *Generalised expectancies for internal versus external control of reinforcement.* Psychological Monographs: General & Applied. 1966; 80 (1): 1-28.

17. Grynderup, M.B. *et al.* 'Work-unit measures of organisational justice and risk of depression – a 2-year cohort study.' *Journal of Occupational and Environmental Medicine* 2013 Jun; 70 (6): 380-5.

18. Grynderup, M.B. *et al.* 'A two-year follow-up study of risk of depression according to work-unit measures of psychological demands and decision latitude.' *Scandinavian Journal of Work, Environment and Health* 2012, Nov 38 (6): 527-36.

THANK YOU

First of all, we would like to thank all of the people who have shown – and continue to show – us so much trust by attending our clinic for treatment or counselling. It is a privilege to be allowed to follow you on your journey, and we are so inspired by our experiences with you.

Regarding the development of stress prevention management, we would particularly like to thank the many managers and employees we have had the pleasure of teaching and consulting, both one-to-one and on individual courses. Your descriptions and experiences enabled us to gain insight into the challenges and dilemmas presented in this book.

We would also like to thank our current and former employees for their hard work and the thoughts and ideas they so willingly shared with us. Many of the book's points emerged from our daily conversations and collaboration.

A huge thank you to our partners, from both work and the many projects we have been allowed to be a part of: companies, municipalities and insurance and pension firms.

How one construes an event
causes one's emotional reaction to it.
Aristoteles